Living Confidently with HIV

Blue Stallion Publications
(Part of The Oxford Development Centre)
The Oxford Development Centre
47 High Street
Witney
Oxfordshire
OX28 6JA

www.bluestallion.co.uk
www.oxdev.co.uk

Blue Stallion Publications is committed to publishing high-quality
therapeutic resource books and works in close professional liasion
with The Oxford Stress and Trauma Centre.

Editor: Dr. Claudia Herbert
Cover design: Axel Silberman (www.silbermanndesign.de)
Cover image: © Ruth Davy (www.ruth-davy.co.uk)
Page design: Simon Ryder (www.designbyfontanel.org)

ISBN 978-1-904127-09-3

Printed and bound in Europe

# Living Confidently with HIV

## A SELF-HELP BOOK FOR PEOPLE LIVING WITH HIV

Liz Shaw

Erasmo Tacconelli

Robert Watson

Claudia Herbert

# Rt Hon Lord Smith of Finsbury
## (Chris Smith)

When I was first diagnosed with HIV, over twenty-two years ago now, I assumed that I was going to die very soon. At the time, very little was known about HIV and the things it could lead to. There was no therapy or treatment available. And too many people had already died. I remember one of the things my doctor said to me: "You are going to have to learn to live with uncertainty"; and to an extent that remains true, as none of us really know what the future will bring. But there have been huge advances in medical knowledge and science since then.

The advent of combination therapy has transformed the picture and the prognosis, and has effectively turned a terminal illness into a manageable chronic condition. It's still not a bundle of fun, being HIV positive. You have to remember constantly to take the medication. There is still discrimination. There are side-effects. The uncertainty hasn't vanished. But for twenty-two years I've survived, have led an incredibly active life, and am still pretty healthy and well. Back in 1987 I wouldn't have dreamed that would be possible.

When I talked publicly for the first time about my HIV status, a few years ago, I wanted to emphasise two things. The first was that it is perfectly possible to live well and usefully with HIV – and to make a huge contribution to society in the process. And the second was that I had the benefit of the highest quality of care, monitoring and medication through the NHS. There are millions of people with HIV around the world who are nowhere near as fortunate, and we need to continue to campaign for them to have the access to care and treatment in the same way that we do here.

# Forewords

In the mean time, however, this book is an invaluable manual for those who have HIV or are close to someone who does. It explains with real clarity what the disease is and what it means for someone caught up by it. It sets out the medical responses, the relationships with doctors and the health care system, the ways in which you can be determined to live well, and perhaps above all the emotional strength that can come if you seek it. It's a book of self-help and self-understanding. It will provide comfort, guidance, courage, and confidence where they are very much needed. It is in a very real sense life-affirming.

## Memory Sachikonye
### (i-Base, UKCAB Co-ordinator)

Being told I was HIV positive in January 2002 has been the hardest thing I've had to deal with - and I have come a long way to be living well with it. Having access to up to date clear information from Living Confidently with HIV will be of enormous help in trying to put things into perspective. Good news or bad, having information has been one of the biggest factors in helping me get through this.

I was in control of my life, but that all seemed to fall apart when the news finally sank in. What would my only son, family and friends say and feel? Having to cope with an HIV diagnosis in a foreign country is not easy, especially when every HIV positive person, or rather someone with AIDS, as the saying used to go in Zimbabwe, had died or would not live for longer than six months. I thought I was going to have a miserable, slow and painful death. How much time would I have?

I accessed support groups and soon found out that HIV positive people, like me, have lots of issues. One of the support groups is

UMOJA. As peers, we all know it is not just about the HIV and taking the medication, there are other stressful issues, such as immigration, family, disclosure, relationships, etc. These issues have an effect on our mental health, adherence, sexual function, acceptance of HIV status and failure to focus on the future. Living Confidently with HIV addresses all these issues and helps the reader on how to cope with the emotions coming from these issues.

Seven years of living with HIV, I have not looked back and I am now involved in the following areas:

Locally:
- Co-ordinator of UMOJA
- Service user rep for the HIV Strategic Forum in Enfield and Haringey
- Service user rep for the Physical Disabilities Board in Enfield
- Committee Member of Staff/Patient Forum at North Middlesex hospital

Nationally:
- Positively Women – volunteer, campaigner
- PozFem Regional Coordinator (national network of Positive Women)
- African HIV Policy Network (AHPN) – HIV champion, public speaker

Internationally:
- Trustee: International Community of Women Living with HIV/AIDS (ICW)

The expertise gained from all this work made me the person I am today. I see myself as an HIV advocate who fights for the rights of those living with HIV. I am vocal and will strive to have our voices heard locally, nationally and internationally.

I will use this book as a guide to empower other women and men, too, on how to deal with any issues around their existence with HIV.

# Forewords

It is my dream to see all HIV positive people, new and old, come out empowered and in control of their own lives after reading and using this book.

HIV is still surrounded by huge stigma, 25 years later on. Stigma not only makes it more difficult for people trying to come to terms with and manage their illness on a personal level, but it also interferes with attempts to fight the AIDS epidemic as a whole.

Living Confidently with HIV is a great book that is easy to read and use, with comprehensive up-to-date information on psychosocial issues and the best advice from those that really care and can talk from experience.

So, a huge thanks to everyone involved in putting this book together. All chapters in the book address issues around being empowered to live confidently with HIV. Without being melodramatic, this book gives hope to all HIV positive people and makes a real difference!

# Liz Shaw
## Consultant Clinical Psychologist

As a Consultant Clinical Psychologist I have a commitment to the field of HIV and Sexual Health Psychology and have been working in the NHS in North London for the last 17 years. I was also the Chair of the Faculty of HIV and Sexual Health of the Division of Clinical Psychology in the British Psychological Society. Alongside my colleagues in the committee we encouraged research, conferences, responded to legislation and created resources to improve the lives of our clients. I am always learning from my clients who themselves have to continuously rise to the challenges of the changing HIV epidemic and how it affects them. In my clinical work I am eclectic using mainly cognitive behavioural, systemic and psychodynamic approaches to help people with their problems. I hope that this book reflects my wish to improve the lives of people with HIV and provides them with positive ways of coping.

# Erasmo Tacconelli
## Chartered Clinical Psychologist

I qualified as a Clinical Psychologist in 2000. Throughout my clinical career I have worked within many types of psychological services. I have worked extensively within the field of Sexual Health and HIV and more recently in Clinical Health Psychology. My duties in Clinical Psychology are broad and include therapeutic interventions, consultation, teaching, research, academic work, service development and supervision. My therapeutic approach is eclectic. Particular areas of interest for me clinically are helping people cope successfully with physical health problems, helping people with intersexuality, transsexuality and sexuality issues, sexual functioning and dysfunction problems. I particularly like empowering people in coping with stigma and discrimination. It has been a pleasure working on this book, as I firmly believe that the concept of living well with HIV needs to be more open and accessible to the public.

## Robert Watson
### Chartered Clinical Psychologist

I am a Chartered Clinical Psychologist with over eight years experience of working in the NHS in Sexual Health and Adult Mental Health settings. In these areas, I have worked as a clinician, supervisor, manager and team leader. I have worked with many people who have felt stuck in their lives, because of HIV and have been struck by the resilience and strength that I have seen many HIV positive people use to overcome problems connected with HIV. In addition to clinical work I have been involved in research, teaching, training, and supervising other professionals in the field of HIV and sexual health. My therapeutic approach draws on cognitive behavioural therapy, systemic therapy, and cognitive-analytic therapy. Through my work in the field, I try to make a contribution to countering the stigma, discrimination, and disempowerment associated with HIV in our society, and improving the quality of life of people affected by HIV.

# Dr Claudia Herbert
## Chartered Consultant Clinical Psychologist

I am a specialist in trauma psychology and, as such, over the past eighteen years have worked with many people who have had to come to terms with the shock of facing a life-threatening illness, including learning about being HIV positive. I know about the enormous pain this confronts people with and the time and many questions it takes to turn things round and move from the victim position, which such news inevitably brings, into a position of personal freedom and empowerment. In both writing and editing this book, I hope to have made a positive contribution to helping people adjust to their HIV diagnosis and live their lives well, confidently and enriched, despite or possibly, because of their chronic condition. I am a Chartered Consultant Clinical Psychologist and a Doctor of Clinical Psychology, a UKCP Registered Cognitive Behavioural Psychotherapist, an EMDR Consultant, an ISST Accredited Schema Therapist and an Associate Member of the British Psychological Society (BPS). I was born in 1960 in Germany and have lived and worked in the United Kingdom since 1981. I am the Founder Director of the Oxford Development Centre, which incorporates Oxfordshire's Independent Psychology Service and The Oxford Stress and Trauma Centre and two other services, which have been in existence since 1997. I present at conferences worldwide and am regularly consulted by the media. Therapeutically, I embed Western scientific understanding with holistic and spiritual healing approaches from Eastern cultures into my practice. I have published three books, a book chapter, an audio book and several academic articles on trauma,

# Acknowledgements

which have been translated into different languages worldwide. I am the editor of other books, including a series of self-help books for adolescents and the book 'Resolving Relationship Difficulties with CBT'. I am a member of the editorial board for The Journal of Behavioural and Cognitive Psychotherapy and hold responsibilities at executive level for a number of national organizations.

## AUTHORS' DEDICATION
This book is dedicated to all those who have lived with HIV.

## ACKNOWLEDGEMENTS

The authors would like to thank those who read scripts of the book and who provided us with suggestions, including our clients, colleagues and members of The British Psychological Society (BPS), Division of Clinical Psychology (DCP), Faculty of Sexual Health and HIV.

# CONTENTS

# Introduction

## THE CHANGING FACE OF HIV

As the number of people in the United Kingdom infected with HIV (Human Immunodeficiency Virus) continues to grow, the introduction of new drug therapies for HIV infection (combination therapies) means that it no longer needs to be seen as a "death sentence", but as an infection that can be controlled in the long-term, similar to diabetes or high blood pressure. As a result, many people taking combination therapies have experienced the halting of their HIV disease progression and returning physical health. Others who were previously diagnosed with AIDS (Acquired Immune Deficiency Syndrome) and had only months to live have also experienced improved physical health and the halting of their AIDS diagnosis.

The scale of recovery in people with AIDS is remarkable. It has been referred to as the "Lazarus Syndrome", named after the biblical character, Lazarus, who was brought back from the dead after four days in his tomb. However, these improvements in treatment have been limited to the developed world. At the time of writing the vast majority of people living in sub-Saharan Africa with HIV infection still do not have access to combination therapies and their illness is poorly controlled and often progresses fast.

## FROM A MEDICAL TO A
## PERSON-CENTRED APPROACH TO HIV

Despite improved treatment and prolonged survival in the Western World, because of drug therapies, people continue to experience stresses because they are HIV positive. Recent research suggests that

# Introduction

levels of psychological distress amongst people with HIV infection have actually increased since the new drug treatments were introduced. Psychological research has also shown that the type of disease or its severity is not the strongest predictor of psychological well-being for those living with a chronic illness. In other words, it takes more than being alive to be happy. Areas of life that are more important for a person's well-being include having a supportive partner and friends, good self-esteem, a job or occupation you like, a nice place to live, a sense of purpose or meaning to life, a satisfying sex life, and being able to enjoy yourself.

Our experience of working with people affected by HIV has shown us that HIV can really get in the way of achieving satisfaction in some of these areas of life. Therefore it can really affect people's quality of life. We know how devastating and overwhelming it can be to find out about a diagnosis of HIV and how much it can shatter a person's plans and previously positive outlook on life. Further, while the medical needs may be well catered for, you may feel that little attention is given to your emotional needs and the distress and despair that you may feel.

We have helped many clients who are HIV positive at various points of their HIV cycle. During our work we have discovered that very little written material exists, which could inform and support people who are adjusting to their diagnosis of HIV. We therefore felt that there was a great need for a book that introduces some key themes and ways of dealing with HIV-related issues. We hope that our book will be a useful resource to you, which helps to address some of your own concerns and emotional needs so that you can achieve a more positive way of coping with HIV.

We have also met many people who are HIV positive who have continued to have a good quality of life. These people have rediscovered ways of having a life that feels worth living in spite of having HIV infection. Our experience tells us that everyone has their own unique story to tell about HIV and there are also shared issues, challenges, and dilemmas. We would like to share with you in this book aspects and strategies that have helped other people to live more confidently with HIV and hope that some of these may be helpful and relevant to you, too.

# Aims
# of this book

# Aims of the book

## WHY THE BOOK WAS WRITTEN

As Clinical Psychologists in the fields of Sexual Health and HIV, and Stress and Trauma, we have put this self-help book together based on our clinical, research and service experiences.

Primarily, this book aims to talk frankly about the issues that people with HIV experience face. As HIV is associated with much fear and stigma, this self-help book covers aspects of living with HIV that may be difficult for you to discuss with others. Fear of talking about HIV and HIV disclosure is a problem for many. We hope that this book will help to release some of your fear and work towards lifting some of the stigma that you may also be experiencing.

## WHO IS THIS SELF-HELP BOOK FOR?

This book is aimed at all adults living with HIV and people who would like to help and understand them. It is especially written for those who may experience issues of coming to terms with and adapting to having HIV, including:

- People who are experiencing difficulties accepting their diagnosis or experiencing problems in adjusting to HIV and finding a way forward in their lives.
- People who have health problems, which interfere with their ability to achieve their goals and who are unsure whether they can cope with the demands facing them.
- People who are concerned about the effects of stress on their health and HIV progression.

# Aims of this book

- People who are isolated in their experience of HIV;
  have limited social supports and are concerned about
  talking openly to others about having HIV.
- People who are overwhelmed by emotions resulting
  from having HIV and are not sure on how to cope.
- People who are able to identify specific changes they would
  like to make in their lives consequent to having HIV or those
  who have problems that they want to solve in relation to having
  HIV or some other aspect of their lives, which they no longer
  feel able to pursue but that they would like to re-engage in.
- People who need to find new meanings to living as a
  result of having HIV, and who would like to enhance their
  sense of living for a future and making future plans.
- Partners, carers, family or friends who would like to
  understand more of the issues facing people with
  HIV and how they can support and help them.

As all people living with HIV are different, this book is written for a wide readership and provides general ideas that we hope will be useful for you. You may already be familiar with some of the information we share, but we do hope that there are also some aspects that will be new and helpful to you and others close to or caring for you.

## WHAT CAN THIS BOOK HELP ACHIEVE?

This book can assist you in thinking about helpful ways to live with HIV. We hope that this book can go some way to helping you achieve one or a few of the following:

# Aims of the book

- Increased knowledge about HIV
- Better adjustment to having HIV
- Enhanced confidence in yourself despite having HIV
- Good relationships despite having HIV
- Increased life choices despite having HIV
- Widened support networks
- An improved quality of life with HIV
- A more positive outlook and motivation for the future

In summary, this self-help book is aimed at addressing some of the psychological needs of people who are HIV positive. It answers frequently asked questions and it draws on our clinical experience of what has helped others with HIV. We hope that the book normalises the experience of living with HIV, creates hope for change and provides a way of learning new skills for readers.

In order to make this book relevant and useful for you, we have included 'check-in' times at regular intervals in the book. There are a number of monitoring sheets throughout this book, which are designed to help you check in and assess where you are with regards to particular aspects or feelings relating to your life with HIV.

When feelings are uncomfortable it is human to want to push them aside and not to want to think about them, because of the distress they may cause you. However, our experience has shown that not thinking about them or pushing them out of your mind doesn't make them go away or make them better. Rather the opposite usually happens. They can get stronger and feel even more overwhelming and out of your control. The purpose of the check-in and monitoring opportunities, which we offer in this book, is to help you to become more conscious and aware of the various issues and feelings facing you. This can

# Aims of this book

help you feel more actively in control, rather than overwhelmed. The monitoring sheets are not meant to be prescriptive or like exercises that may remind you of school. Instead they are meant to be interactive and we would like to encourage you to use these, as they seem relevant and helpful to your particular experiences, situation and needs. You may even find it helpful to start a special notebook or diary, which you use solely for the purpose of helping you gain awareness and control over your condition.

How
this

## WHAT IS SELF-HELP

Self-help involves using materials, either alone or with assistance, which are designed to teach new skills and ultimately help you overcome a problem. It is a popular approach and most bookshops have large sections devoted to self-help. Publications cover a range of problems and incorporate a wide variety of methods for tackling these problems. Materials can come in many different forms, including books, tapes, computer programmes and so on.

## ADVANTAGES AND DISADVANTAGES OF SELF-HELP

The advantages of self-help are many. It can be used in your own time. You can work at your own pace so that you can stop, think and reflect on what you are working on. The material will always be available to use at any time and can be reused if at a later stage the problem recurs. A key advantage is that if people are allowed to address their problems themselves, they can feel a real sense of achievement, which may help them also to address other problems in the same way in the future.

However, self-help is not suitable for everyone and all problems. Some people are too unwell to be able to help themselves. For example, concentration problems that often accompany depression may make it difficult for them to retain and practice the information. This may result in a person feeling frustrated as the strategies they attempt might not work. This, in turn, could worsen a person's depression due to added feelings of blame or inadequacy. Some people need professional advice or more intensive approaches, which self-help alone does not provide. If you feel that the latter would apply to you, we would advice that you seek additional professional help, tailored to your individual needs. Nevertheless, this book could still be helpful for you to use alongside the professional help you are receiving.

## WHAT ARE COGNITIVE AND BEHAVIOURAL PSYCHOLOGICAL APPROACHES?

The predominant approaches used in this book are cognitive and behavioural. Put simply, this means that the approaches help you to focus on and understand your thoughts, feelings and behaviours and the links between them. By understanding the links, goals and strategies can then be devised to assist you in overcoming problems.

## THE COPING PROCESS: HOW TO USE THE COPING STRATEGIES IN THIS BOOK

How well you adjust to HIV can be explained in part by your individual way of coping, also called your coping response. The term "coping" refers to the cognitive (thinking), behavioural (doing) and emotional (feeling) strategies that people use to manage stressful situations. This self-help book is filled with various ideas and strategies that others have found helpful in negotiating the particular demands around living with HIV. We use regular check-in boxes throughout the various chapters of this book, which are designed for you to use as reflection time. These will help you personalize the different issues, which are covered in this book. You could use these as you go along, or you might use them entirely independently, checking-in whenever it feels relevant and important to you. You can also use some of the check-in boxes at different times as the issues that you are facing change.

Our understanding of coping in this book is based on the ideas of two psychologists, Lazarus and Folkman (1984). They found that the quality of a person's coping response is determined by both the degree of threat that is posed by an illness and the resources that the person has available to help them cope in the situation. Coping responses are divided into emotion-focused and problem-focused strategies.

There are 11 chapters in this book, which is divided into three parts: *Part A: Living Confidently with HIV* covers basic information and advice on key aspects of living with HIV; *Part B: Emotion-focussed Strategies* and *Part C: Problem-focussed Strategies* cover specific techniques and ideas for coping with a variety of emotionally demanding and challenging HIV-related issues. Each chapter provides insights, perspectives and strategies to address that particular issue.

The coping strategies people use to tackle problems associated with HIV infection partly explains how well they adapt to living with the condition. This book contains a range of strategies that can help you deal with difficulties that may arise. The type of strategy you use will depend on the problem you are facing. In this section we explain how to select the most appropriate strategies.

## PART A: LIVING CONFIDENTLY WITH HIV

Within Part A, there are numerous coping strategies put forward, relating to various aspects of living with HIV covered in each chapter.

From Chapters one to five the approaches suggested are educative and strategic. The topics covered include:

- Understanding what HIV is
- Being more health aware
- Being more in control of your health and social network
- Increasing your confidence about disclosure
- Feeling more confident with close and/or sexual relationships.

## PART B: EMOTION-FOCUSED STRATEGIES & PART C: PROBLEM-FOCUSED STRATEGIES

Parts B and C are divided into emotion-focused and problem-focused strategies. The purpose of emotion-focused coping is to manage emotions associated with stressful situations. The purpose of problem-focused coping is to actively do something to alter or change the problem situation. Research has shown that both emotion-focused and problem-focused strategies can be useful depending on the situation people are facing. The most important factor to consider when deciding what type of strategies to use is the degree to which the situation causing stress is controllable or changeable.

Problem-focused strategies are more useful when it is reasonably clear that something can be done to change the situation, which is causing you stress. Examples are working out how to attend a HIV voluntary sector organisation to combat loneliness, using techniques to specifically address anxiety and depression symptoms, obtaining alternative therapies to alleviate side-effects of medication, or attending a course to increase your sense of purpose in life and so on.

Conversely when little can be done to alter the situation, which is causing stress, acceptance and emotion-focused strategies will be more useful. Examples are accepting your own emotional responses to a relationship ending as valid, talking to someone about your emotions associated with being diagnosed HIV positive, or using mindfulness techniques to feel calm if you are nervous awaiting test results.

You may find yourself needing to use both types of strategies for different aspects of the same problem.

The decision tree on the next page can be useful to start you thinking about how to help yourself by using Part B and Part C of this book. Use the decision tree to help you decide which chapters and coping strategies you wish to use. Remember that different strategies help at different times. Therefore, picking the one that you feel is right for you at a given time is the best way forward. If you are not sure what your particular issues are, Part A will help you begin to think of the areas of your life that it may be helpful for you to address.

**SITUATION**

Examples include:

Accepting being HIV+

Learning about HIV

Coping with your emotions

Disclosing your HIV status

Reducing stress

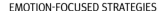

"Is my problem controllale and open to change?"

NO

YES

**EMOTION-FOCUSED STRATEGIES**

Chapter 6: Understanding HIV-Associated Emotions

Chapter 7: When Emotions are Difficult

Chapter 8: Mindfulness and HIV

**PROBLEM-FOCUSED STRATEGIES**

Chapter 9: Anxiety and Depression Strategies

Chapter 10: Problem-solving

Chapter 11: Visualising the Future

LIVING CONFIDENTLY WITH HIV

EMOTION-FOCUSED STRATEGIES

PROBLEM-FOCUSED STRATEGIES

# 1

Diagnosed HIV Positive (HIV+)

# INTRODUCTION

Having a diagnosis of HIV can change your life in many ways. This makes it important to be able to adjust to living with it. Fortunately, many people with HIV are able to live long and fulfilling lives now, because of the medical treatments available. Because of this we can now pay attention to what "Living with HIV" actually means for a person with an HIV diagnosis.

HIV is well known for the emotional reactions that it produces. The fact that people believed (and some may still believe), that you could catch it from someone by sharing cutlery or the toilet, just illustrates the extent of misunderstanding surrounding HIV. Therefore, the better your knowledge about your condition, the better will be your ability to deal with your own and other people's emotional reactions.

This chapter will explain the health improvements in HIV as a result of the new drug treatments and how they may impact upon you. The ideas put forward will provide a basis upon which the rest of this book will refer to.

The key point of this chapter is that the more you understand your condition the more in control you will feel in your life.

PART
A

PART
B

PART
C

# WHAT IS HIV?

Human Immunodeficiency Virus (HIV) still has the potential to weaken the immune system despite improved prognosis as a result of the drugs. HIV is a virus that attacks the immune system, which is the body's defence against disease. If not stopped HIV can then cause Acquired Immune Deficiency Syndrome (AIDS). This is the name given to a group of medical conditions, which may develop when HIV has damaged a person's immune system.

The word used to predict the probable course of a disease is 'prognosis'. This comes from an ancient Greek word meaning 'to know beforehand'. It is the terminal prognosis associated with HIV that has caused so much concern. When HIV emerged in the population in the early 1980's there was much fear. This was largely due to the fact that there was no cure and that many people died shortly following the onset of illness. Although, there is still no cure in terms of reversing or completely healing HIV at the moment, people now can live with HIV for many years. Therefore HIV has changed from being seen as a terminal condition to being seen as a chronic condition.

PART
A

PART
B

PART
C

# HOW HAS HIV BECOME A CHRONIC CONDITION?

The shift in prognosis from terminal to chronic shown in Figure (1) is due to the use of Highly Active Antiretroviral Therapy (HAART), the new drug therapy we refer to, which slows the rate at which HIV reproduces.

As increased life expectancy simply means more time to live, there is now, more than ever, a need to focus on and attend to 'living with HIV'. Living can be difficult at times though, and there are extra issues for those who are HIV positive. Adjusting to HIV requires understanding what has changed and what hasn't. Attention to particular issues of concern may make living easier and far more worthwhile.

To capture this change from terminal to chronic, and the specific HIV-related issues that occur, also look at Figure (2): Before HAART, (before the new HIV drugs were available) and Figure (3): After HAART, (after

**HIV as a TERMINAL ILLNESS**
A person diagnosed HIV+ in the early 1990's would know that death was largely inevitable. HIV, during this time, led to AIDS, which was a terminal illness. Only health consequences could be medically managed, such as infections resulting from low immunity.

**HIV as a CHRONIC CONDITION**
A person diagnosed HIV+ in the late 1990's and after, knows that death is not necessarily inevitable, because of HIV antiretroviral drugs. HIV is now a chronic condition, which can be managed, instead of inevitably progressing to AIDS. Thus life expectancy is considerably prolonged.

PART
A

PART
B

PART
C

**Fig. 1** From terminal to chronic illness

the new HIV drugs were available) presented further on. This is a way of understanding the life cycle of HIV and the issues you may encounter.

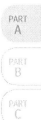 **SELF-MONITORING: A CHANCE TO CHECK-IN WITH YOURSELF** ▪ *terminal to chronic ( 1 ) Based on Fig. 1, what were your thoughts? Does it make sense to you that HIV can be both a terminal illness and a chronic condition? (2) What does having a manageable condition mean to you? Check-in with yourself to reflect on what the issues are facing you right now? It could be*

*very helpful to make some notes about the above in your diary,
notebook or on a sheet of paper, so that you can later decide on
what might help you to take some of your observations further.*

# WHEN ANTIRETROVIRALS
# ARE NOT AVAILABLE

Figure (2) shows the course of HIV before the new HIV drugs were
available (or in countries where they are still unavailable). It can be seen
from this figure that a series of stages are progressed through, leading
to health decline.

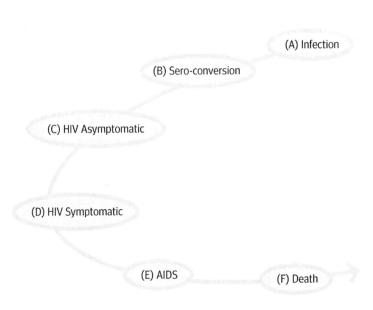

**Fig. 2** Before HAART (Late 1980s to Early 1990s)

* (A) INFECTION: at the infection stage, the main routes of transmission are unprotected sexual intercourse, intravenous drug use, and vertical transmission (the transmission of the virus within the HIV+ pregnant woman to her growing foetus). It takes some time for the virus to build up in the body and be detected by HIV blood testing.

* (B) SERO-CONVERSION: When the virus is detectable on testing at around three months after infection, a person is said to have "sero-converted". This period is sometimes called the "window period".

* (C) HIV ASYMPTOMATIC: The virus continues to reproduce and stage C is reached, namely that the person is HIV+ but has no symptoms.

* (D) HIV SYMPTOMATIC: With time, the virus reproduces leading to the development of symptoms at stage D. As the immune system or body defence system is weakened, symptoms can develop such as oral thrush, fatigue, night sweats or skin conditions.

* (E) AIDS: The virus then continues to reproduce and progresses to the Acquired Immune Deficiency Syndrome (AIDS) stage at which point opportunistic infections (infections that take advantage of a weakened immune system) might develop. These infections could develop in the form of pneumocystus carinii (PCP, pneumonia), cytomegalovirus (CMV, a virus that causes blindness), Tuberculosis (TB), and a variety of cancers, including karposi sarcoma that generally affects the skin. In the past, all the medicines that were available treated only the symptoms of these opportunistic infections. The virus itself, which compromised the immune system and, which was responsible for these opportunistic infections, could not be reached and controlled in any way.

* (F) DEATH: In this stage the virus has replicated sufficiently to damage the immune system. As a result the body will be unable to fight the arising opportunistic infections leading to death.

PART
A

PART
B

PART
C

# AFTER THE AVAILABILITY OF ANTIRETROVIRALS

In contrast, Figure (3) shows the course of HIV when the new HIV treatments are available. The main tests to assess the course of the illness are now the "CD4 T-cell" and the "Viral Load" (VL) blood counts. The "CD4 T-cell" blood counts give an indication of the health of the immune system and the "Viral Load" (VL) blood counts look at the amount of HIV in the blood. These are usually carried out every three to six months. Generally speaking, if your CD4 count falls and the VL increases the risk of becoming unwell becomes higher.

The good news is that people with the virus are living much longer now. At the present time the exact long-term prognosis is unclear, since effective treatment has only been available since 1996. However, many health professionals involved in HIV care are very optimistic about long-term prognosis and health outcomes. This is similar to other areas of medicine, such as the change in prognosis associated with diabetes, following the discovery of insulin. However, currently there is still no cure for HIV infection.

## Stages A to F

In Figure 3 the development of the virus to AIDS (A to F) can still occur, because it is not the virus that has changed but its management. A person can still be diagnosed at any stage after seroconversion. AIDS, or a $CD_4$ count of less than 200, means that the individual is still increasingly susceptible to a host of opportunistic infections and cancers.

The majority of people when prescribed HAART, find that the virus slows down its reproduction and therefore halts any disease progression. Most people find that their health improves and many report undetectable viral loads (where there are not enough HIV particles in a blood sample for the viral load test to count. This does not mean, however, that you do not have HIV in your body).

## Stage G

At this stage, if HAART is well adhered to, HIV spread and its consequences may be held in check. For the HIV positive person this is the stage to aim to remain at.

While on HAART many clients find that they do remain there and do not progress to stages D, E and F. They are still HIV+ but the virus is well controlled. This is illustrated diagrammatically in Figure (3), where HAART is represented as a barrier to HIV progression.

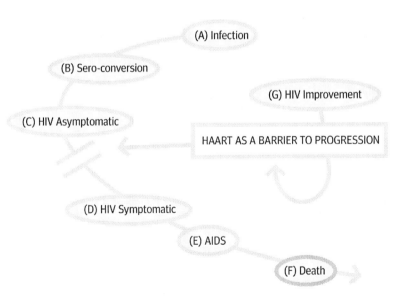

Fig. 3 After HAART (Late 1990s to Present Day)

A useful way of understanding this is to imagine making popcorn. When the heat in the pan increases and makes the corn pop, the lid keeps the popping corn in. It is safely contained. But if the lid is removed (the drugs are not taken) the popcorn gets out and spreads all over.

# WHAT TO EXPECT FROM LIVING WITH THE CHRONIC CONDITION OF HIV?

PART
A

PART
B

PART
C

Despite improved treatments you may well still feel your health is vulnerable and that HIV could drastically shorten your life. This is an entirely understandable reaction, especially given the past history of HIV, as outlined earlier, and the resulting images that may have been created in people's minds.

The previous diagrams demonstrated the changes in health status and how health improvement can be achieved, despite a diagnosis of HIV. We now propose a psychological model of HIV. This will explain to you the so-called "pendulum of uncertainty" that you may find yourself experiencing when living with HIV.

# THE FOUR PHASES OF HIV

Figure (4) shows four phases that encapsulate the issues a person with HIV may confront. The first is the *Risk Phase* during which infection may take place. Infection with HIV will then lead to the *Diagnosis Phase*. Following that, a person will either be at the *Latent Phase* or the *Manifest Phase*. This will depend on the extent to which HIV has

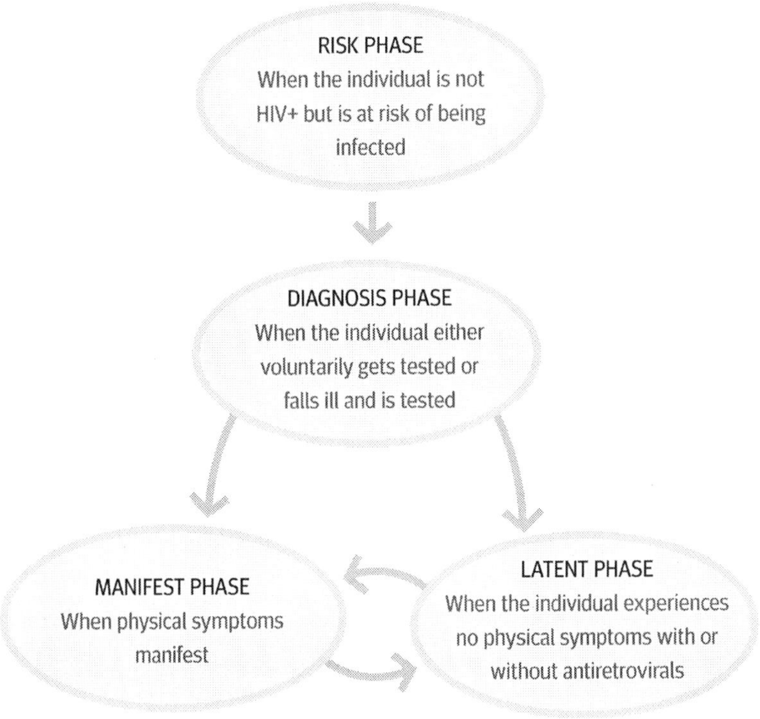

**RISK PHASE**
When the individual is not
HIV+ but is at risk of being
infected

**DIAGNOSIS PHASE**
When the individual either
voluntarily gets tested or
falls ill and is tested

**MANIFEST PHASE**
When physical symptoms
manifest

**LATENT PHASE**
When the individual experiences
no physical symptoms with or
without antiretrovirals

PART
A

PART
B

PART
C

Fig. 4 The 4 Phases of HIV

increased in the body, on the symptoms that manifest and ultimately on the efficacy of the combination of antiretroviral drugs prescribed.

However, a person can oscillate between the Latent Phase and the Manifest Phase. This can be imagined like a 'pendulum of uncertainty', because it is the uncertainty that becomes a central experience for people living with HIV. This uncertainty can have its origin in many areas. There is, for example, uncertainty relating to the medical issues of HIV. People can be faced with ambiguous symptoms, complex treatments and their side effects and the unpredictable course of the disease for each individual. There can also be uncertainty surrounding personal issues, such as changes in a person's felt identity, in their close personal relationship with their living partner or relatives, in their ability to maintain work and their financial status. Another area of uncertainty when living with HIV can relate to people's social life, for example, the unpredictable reactions from others or changes in the friendship network.

Every person's journey will be different and will depend upon many interrelated factors. Depending on these, you may find that you experience different amounts of uncertainty at different stages and times, while living with HIV. Even though uncomfortable at times, it can be tremendously helpful for you to recognize which experiences are contributing to your feelings of uncertainty at any one time. This in itself may enable you to start to feel in greater control of your illness.

PART
A

PART
B

PART
C

## IMPORTANT QUESTIONS AT EACH PHASE

To help you think about your own issues, the following boxes in Figure (5) contain the four phases with quotes to illustrate common experiences and questions that people with HIV may face. It is common for many different issues to arise, some will be specific to a particular phase of the illness and others may be relevant throughout all phases. Before HAART these were largely related to thinking about death. Now, after HAART, they are about treatments, their side effects and the future.

At present, for example, a person at the 'Diagnosis Phase' will be faced with many adjustments due to the expected changes in health and life style that may lie ahead. A person at the 'Manifest Phase' may

## QUESTIONS at the RISK PHASE
### WHEN THE INDIVIDUAL IS NOT HIV+ BUT IS AT RISK
### OF BEING INFECTED

"How might I get HIV?" • "Am I a risk or at risk?" • "I forgot to have safe sex – what will the consequences be for me?" • "I was forced to have unprotected sex against my will, am I HIV positive?" • "Is my sexual practice safe?" • "Why am I too scared to tell my partner to use a condom?" • "I will never get HIV as I am not in an at risk group... or am I?" • "I don't have to worry about safe sex, I know my partner is faithful... or isn't s/he?"

## QUESTIONS at the DIAGNOSIS PHASE
### WHEN THE INDIVIDUAL VOLUNTARILY GETS TESTED OR
### FALLS ILL AND IS TESTED

"Where did I get it from?" • "How long do I have left to live?" • "Who shall I tell... should I tell?" • "Will I be judged or blamed for this by others, forever?" • "How do I possibly tell others?" • "I can't believe this has happened – will I ever come to terms with this?" • "What am I going to do – my life is changed forever?" • "Is my life still worth living?" • "What will happen to me?"

## QUESTIONS at the MANIFEST PHASE
### WHEN PHYSICAL SYMPTOMS MANIFEST

"Shall I start combination therapy?" • "Am I taking my medicines properly?" • "Does the treatment work for me?" • "Do I need another combination of drugs?" • "Will I get better?" • "Will I have to make changes to my life due to my current ill-health?" • "Will my new combination make me feel better again?" • "Will I get side effects?" • "How do I deal with the responses toward me from others now that I show symptoms?"

**Fig. 5** Important HIV-related Questions

PART
A

PART
B

PART
C

need to consider different treatment options and their side effects. A person at the 'Latent Phase' may experience undetectable viral loads, but may have treatment side effects. Do some of the questions, below, seem familiar to you?

We hope that if you experience any of these thoughts, you will find some of the answers and coping suggestions in this book helpful to you.

**SELF-MONITORING: A CHANCE TO CHECK-IN WITH YOURSELF** • *HIV phases (1) Based on the 'After HAART' diagram in Figure (3) allow yourself some time to work out, which HIV phase you are finding yourself in at the moment? (2) Following this, you might like to check-in with yourself to reflect on the issues that this brings up for you and the implications of this that you are facing right now? It could be very helpful to make some notes about the above in your diary, notebook or on a sheet of paper, so that you can later decide on what might help you to take some of your observations further.*

PART
A

PART
B

PART
C

# CONCLUSION

It takes time for people to understand a complex health condition like HIV. When you were diagnosed, you probably found it very difficult to take in any information at such an emotionally challenging time. You may have been too overwhelmed and pre-occupied with your initial emotional reactions to HIV to be able to really understand what HIV actually is. We hope that so far the book has helped you to understand HIV a little better. This is important because faulty, inaccurate or incomplete beliefs will get in the way of the natural psychological adjustment process that is so important for you to achieve in order for you to be able to live more positively with HIV.

We will address the issues and dilemmas in each of the four phases discussed in the course of this book. Everyone adjusts to HIV in their own way, because every person is unique and their circumstances are different. We encourage you to not compare yourself with others, as this could put you into an unfair evaluation. We believe that it is far more helpful for you to recognize and accept the issues surrounding your particular circumstances, as this will enable you to respond to and make changes where possible.

PART
A

PART
B

PART
C

# 2

Health, Stress and Lifestyles

# INTRODUCTION

In this chapter we concentrate on the lifestyle you adopt and how this is important to living with HIV. If you switch on the television, open a newspaper or visit your HIV clinic or General Practitioner, you usually don't have to look far to find some advice on lifestyle issues, such as diet, exercise, smoking or alcohol. Sometimes the amount of health advice available can seem bewildering and this can make it hard for people to make lifestyle choices that feel right for them. What we would like to suggest to you is that we now know from the field of Psycho-immunology, which is the study of the effects of psychological factors on your immune system, that stress relating to lifestyle factors is linked to HIV disease progression. This means that the more stress a person experiences as a result of an unhelpful lifestyle, the greater the negative effect on the way their HIV is likely to progress. In this chapter we explain how we understand stress, and provide you with some ideas on how to manage stresses when they arise in your life. Everyone feels stressed at some point in his or her life, and this can affect your quality of life. Being aware of what you can do to minimise your levels of stress and to look after your body, can help you stay well while living with HIV.

PART
A

PART
B

PART
C

# WHAT IS STRESS?

We have all, at some point in our lives, felt stressed about a problem we have faced, and it is usually because we can't see a way of dealing with it. This can leave us feeling stuck and overwhelmed. Common effects of stress are anxiety, depression, anger, irritability or exhaustion.

The stress response of your body is rather like an aeroplane taking off down a runway. Virtually all systems (such as, the heart and blood vessels, the immune system, the lungs, the digestive system, the sensory organs and brain) are activated and working at full power to respond to what you may perceive as a threat or danger in some form. Stress involves the entire human system and consumes a lot of energy. Continuous stress can make you feel very drained.

There are many things that can cause us to feel "stressed out". These can include situations we find ourselves in, such as, for example, work, our living environment, our finances; but also the way, in which we think about ourselves, the people around us, the world and our future.

Stress is the result of an imbalance between the demands made on our personal resources, both by the outside world and by us, and our ability to deal with these demands. Figure (6) shows the relationship between resources and demands. The balance between a person's resources and the demands being made on them can be compared with a bank account. If too many demands are made on the account we go into the 'red' and become overdrawn, which is comparable to being under stress. Under normal circumstances we can cope with the everyday demands of life, such as the maintenance of a job and relationships, which is comparable to the way routine standing orders regularly diminish our financial account. It is only when extra stresses or demands come along that we can tip over 'into the red'. Sometimes, a crisis may be the result of a 'last straw', which just tips the balance and we fall 'into the red', or become stressed.

Therefore, especially when you are affected by physical conditions that can weaken or attack your immune system, such as HIV, it is important to be aware of your stress levels and try to keep your "stress account", just like a bank account, in a positive balance. In order to be able to do so, it can be very helpful for you to become aware of the amount of demands that you are facing in your everyday life and the amount of resources that are available to you to cope with these demands. Awareness of this will enable you to recognize the current status of your stress balance. If you feel that this is in a negative balance or 'in the red', you then have a choice of decreasing the demands that you are facing at this time in your life or increasing the resources that you have available to yourself. This book is designed to support you with this.

PART
A

PART
B

PART
C

1. Demands of everyday life

2. Adjustments to new situations

3. Attitudes and expectations

4. Unexpected circumstances/ill health

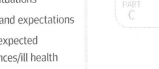

DEMANDS

1. Physical health

2. Skills and experience

3. Attitudes and beliefs

4. Emotional make-up

5. Social support

6. Ability to relax

RESOURCES

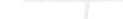

Fig. 6 Balancing Resources with Demands

# ACUTE OR CHRONIC STRESS?

Acute stress is the reaction to an immediate threat, commonly known as the "fight or flight" response. The threat can be any situation that you experience, even subconsciously or falsely, as a danger. Common acute stressors include, noise, crowding, isolation, hunger, danger, infection, and also imagining a threat or remembering a dangerous event. Acute stress initially triggers the release of particular hormones (e.g. norepinephrine, also called adrenaline), which prepare the body and mind to respond to the stress, such as with a fight or flight response. Usually, once the acute threat has passed, the response becomes inactivated and your hormone levels return to normal. This is a condition called the 'relaxation response'. Stress under these circumstances is a normal bodily response, designed to protect the person.

Chronic stress, in comparison, is the long-term reaction to stressors. As modern life poses ongoing stressful situations that are not short-lived, the stress then becomes chronic. Common chronic stressors include, for example, ongoing highly pressured work, long-term relationship problems, ongoing health problems, loneliness and perceived social isolation and persistent financial worries. The latter can lead to a chronic release of the stress hormones, which then is no longer a normal or healthy response and can seriously impact on a person's health.

# NEGATIVE EFFECTS OF STRESS

In the modern world, the stress response can sometimes be an asset for raising levels of performance during critical events, such as, a sports activity, an important meeting, or in situations of actual danger or crisis. If stress, however, becomes persistent and low-level, all parts of the body's stress apparatus, such as the brain, the heart, the lungs, the vessels and the muscles become chronically over- or under-activated. This may produce physical or psychological damage over time.

Stress-related conditions that are most likely to produce negative side effects to a person include the following:

- An accumulation of persistent stressful situations, particularly those that you cannot easily control. This could, for example, be high-pressured work plus an unhappy relationship.
- Persistent stress following a severe acute response to a traumatic event, such as a road traffic accident (RTA) or an assault. This can sometimes lead to a condition, called Posttraumatic Stress Disorder (PTSD), with symptoms such as nightmares, intrusive thoughts and flashbacks about the traumatic events.
- An inefficient or insufficient relaxation response. This would occur if you have never learned to set aside times in which you deliberately induce a relaxation response, by, for example, rushing around all day with no rest.
- Stress can diminish your quality of life by reducing feelings of pleasure and accomplishment. This in itself then can threaten relationships and perpetuate further stress.
- A lowered immune response, due to the blunting of the immune system in response to chronic stress. This, in turn, increases the risk of infections, which, in turn, can then become the cause of further stress.

PART
A

PART
B

PART
C

# WHAT OTHER CONDITIONS HAVE THE SAME SYMPTOMS AS STRESS?

It is important to recognise and identify how you are feeling, both physically and psychologically, so that you are able to differentiate between mood problems and stress, and get the help you need for them. If you know what you are experiencing, you will also be more aware of what you can do to help yourself. Feelings and symptoms, whether they are physical or psychological or both, can be confusing. Below is a summary of how to recognise two of the most common ones occurring in people with HIV: Anxiety and Depression.

## FEATURES OF ANXIETY

The physical symptoms of anxiety mirror many of those of stress, including a fast heart rate, rapid shallow breathing, and, increased muscle tension. Anxiety is an emotional condition, however, and is characterised by feelings of apprehension, uncertainty, fear or panic. These feelings typically correspond to how a person perceives and thinks about particular aspects in their life. However, they do not necessarily correspond to that person's actual circumstances in their current life. Sometimes, they can arise from untreated experiences of chronic stress or even trauma, even relating as far back as to events in a person's childhood.

Therefore, unlike with external triggers for stress, the triggers for anxiety are not necessarily associated with actual, specifically stressful or threatening external conditions. They usually arise internally. Nevertheless, the internal physiological process that occurs in an anxious person's body is the same as it would be for someone actually facing specific external conditions of stress. The body therefore responds to and expresses the emotions that this person is experiencing. Some individuals with anxiety problems have numerous physical complaints, such as headaches, gastrointestinal disturbances, dizziness, and chest pain. Severe anxiety problems can be very debilitating, and can interfere with career, family and social spheres. If this is the case for you, you can obtain a referral to a psychological therapist, such as a Clinical Psychologist or a Psychotherapist, to help you gain understanding of why you have these symptoms and what you might try to overcome them.

## FEATURES OF DEPRESSION

Depression can be a very disabling condition, and, like anxiety disorders, may result from untreated chronic stress or trauma, sometimes relating to current life circumstances, but also often relating to unresolved experiences from the past. Depression also mimics some of the symptoms of stress including: changes in appetite, sleep patterns and concentration.

Serious depression is distinguished from stress by feelings of chronic sadness, hopelessness, loss of interest in life, physical apathy, total lack of motivation and, sometimes, thoughts or actual intentions of suicide. Acute depression is also accompanied by significant changes in functioning. This might include: decreased appetite, sleep problems, concentration and memory problems or worrying negative thoughts. A professional, psychological assessment may be needed in order to determine if depression is caused by stress (secondary to stress) or if it is the primary problem. In either case, if these feelings persist, it may be helpful for a person to pursue a course of psychological therapy. You may also wish to read Chapter 10, which offers you information on further help with these two problems.

PART
A

PART
B

PART
C

# WHAT STRESSORS ARE THERE IN YOUR LIFE?

There are many potential sources of stress for people with HIV. Below, we include for you some examples of what these might be.

## (1) EMOTIONAL STRESSORS

These include fears and anxieties that you may struggle with and may worry about. Every person will have a unique set of these. They could be about diagnosis, what will happen in the course of the illness, about taking your medication, the possible side effects, and about death and dying and the meaning that this carries for you.

## (2) SOCIAL STRESSORS

HIV is a stigmatising disease and many people worry about what judgements other people make with regards to how they contracted it and the effect this may have on their social status. This includes worries about what partners, family, friends and even strangers may think about you. People can become very isolated as a result of these worries. The isolation may be social isolation, but can also include physical isolation, including other people keeping a greater physical distance from you during social contact. This can be an enormous source of stress.

## (3) CHANGE AND UNCERTAINTY

The course your HIV illness takes can be very unsettling to you, because it may involve losses and changes that you have to go through. Depending on what these are, you may find yourself feeling more or less in control over these. This can include getting used to having the virus and what it means for your life, changes to your life plans, loosing previously important relationships, stopping or changing work, dealing with symptoms and opportunistic infections, changing your habits to more healthy ones, and taking medication.

## (4) CHEMICAL STRESSORS

Some people turn to drugs and alcohol in order to cope, which puts a further stress on their body. Some of the medication you may take to help control your condition of HIV may also cause you side effects, which can be very stressful. Sometimes people turn to non-prescription drugs or alcohol as a means of coping with these. If this applies to you, you may need to find ways of coping with the side effects differently, especially if they last for a while or recur.

## (5) DECISION STRESSORS

Throughout the course of your condition there will be many decisions to be taken.

These include:

* as to whether you wish to be tested in the first place
* whom you tell about your diagnosis
* when to start combination therapies
* which drugs to take and many others, which may cause you stress.

The stress is caused by the recognition that whatever decision you take, there will be certain consequences and sometimes costs attached to them. The difficulty is that many of the consequences of your decisions cannot be known beforehand, which therefore can make it feel very stressful for you to decide.

PART A

PART B

PART C

## (6) DISEASE STRESSORS

HIV is a chronic condition, which may potentially take a long course. During this, you may be facing many possible physical consequences, such as opportunistic infections, treatments and their effects on the body, such as physical pain or discomfort, possible changes in appearance and understandable worries about these. It is difficult to plan for the physical consequences that you may be encountering, as these vary greatly in terms of type, severity, frequency and time of occurrence between each person. Therefore, stress may be caused both by the nature of the actual physical consequences, as well as, by their unpredictability and your inability to plan for these.

## (7) ENVIRONMENTAL STRESSORS

Contracting HIV leads to significant changes in your life circumstances and can have considerable consequences on factors in your environment. For example, you may find that there is an increased uncertainty regarding your finances, housing and relationships. These changes in environmental circumstances can be upsetting and very stressful to you.

In addition to the above stressors that are more specific to HIV, there will be the usual life events that may put further stress on you, such as pregnancy, the ending of relationships unrelated to HIV, arguments and conflict, moving house, challenges in terms of your work or occupational path, societal or cultural struggles and other major life event changes.

The self-monitoring instructions, opposite, will provide you with an opportunity to evaluate which stressors are currently affecting your life. This in turn, may enable you to make some necessary changes or tackle the stressors differently.

SELF-MONITORING: A CHANCE TO CHECK-IN WITH YOURSELF • *Anxiety, depression and stress* ( I ) *Based on the descriptions of anxiety, depression and stress, allow yourself some time to work out whether you experience any of these feelings at the moment? How do these feelings express themselves in your life? (2) You might then like to check-in with yourself to reflect on the stressors existing in your present life. It could be very helpful to make some notes about the above in your diary, notebook or on a sheet of paper, so that you can later decide on what might help you to take some of your observations further.*

# COGNITIVE-BEHAVIOURAL STRESS REDUCTION TECHNIQUES

PART
A

PART
B

PART
C

We have suggested that a helpful start to enhancing a healthy lifestyle with HIV is to reduce stress. You may now like to try the following methods taken from Cognitive Behavioural Therapy (CBT) that have been found to be effective ways to help reduce stress. These include: identifying the sources of stress, restructuring your priorities, changing your response to stress, and finding methods for managing and reducing the stressors in your life. This approach is particularly helpful when the source of stress is chronic.

## STEP (1): IDENTIFYING SOURCES OF STRESS
Can you identify, which sources of stress apply to you from the list of potential stressors, outlined above? There may be others, not listed here, which apply to you. It would be helpful for you to make a list of all the sources of stress that you can identify in your current life.

You can then use this list in conjunction with the check-in given on the previous page.

- It is useful to start the process of stress reduction with a diary that keeps an informal inventory of daily activities and events. This task does not have to be done in great detail. A few words accompanying a time and date will usually be enough to serve to remind you of the particular event or activity.
- Then note activities that put a strain on your energy and time, trigger anger or anxiety, or precipitate a negative physical response, such as an upset stomach or headache.
- Also note positive experiences, such as, those that are mentally or physically refreshing or produce a sense of accomplishment or give you pleasure or joy.
- After a week or two, you can try to identify two or three events or activities that have been significantly upsetting or overwhelming. You may even give them a rating in terms of how stressful they have been for you on a rating scale between 0 and a 100 (where 0 = no stress at all, and 100 = exceedingly stressful)

## STEP (2): QUESTIONING THE SOURCES OF STRESS

You can then ask yourself the following questions:

- Are you doing these stressful activities for yourself or someone else? If you have done them for someone else, you might like to understand what makes you take on extra responsibilities during a time when you may not have the resource to spare?
- Have you taken on tasks that are not manageable?
- Which tasks are in your control and which aren't?

PART
A

PART
B

PART
C

- Can you change anything about them to make them less stressful?
- Do you enjoy what you are doing?
- Do you value what you are doing?

## STEP (3): RESTRUCTURING PRIORITIES

The next step you may like to try is to attempt to shift the balance from stress producing to stress reducing activities. Eliminating stress is rarely practical or feasible, but there are many ways to reduce its impact:

- **Reduce the priority of activities in your life that are unhelpful.**
  For example, by not avoiding people because you are afraid of what they might think if they knew your status. This would help you to develop more social support and face your fears. You may find it helpful to be aware of your own patterns of wanting to help or rescue others. In order to reduce the impact of stress it will be important for you to establish contact with people, with whom you can have a reciprocal relationship rather than feeling that you have to be the one who has to take on even more caring. This may be a good opportunity to explore the criteria by which you normally choose friends and it may help you to be more conscious of your patterns and you could choose to engage in healthy and equal relationships.
- **Make time for recreation and breaks.** This may be a good opportunity for you to explore, what is preventing you from giving yourself time for recreation. Notice how you feel when you give yourself breaks. Is it something that comes easy to you or is it something that induces guilt? Allow yourself to notice any self-defeating behaviour or unhelpful response patterns. This may be a good opportunity to start to challenge some of your unhelpful thoughts about yourself in relation to taking time for recreation and breaks.

PART
A

PART
B

PART
C

- **Replace unnecessary time consuming chores with pleasurable or interesting activities.** Notice any thoughts or internal dialogues in yourself that may tell you that you 'should' be doing chores before you have fun or that may forbid you to have fun or pleasure at all. There may also be a part of you that feels that somehow you are to blame for your condition and that may want to punish you by now depriving you of any pleasure. Allow yourself to look closely at some of your internal patterns. This may be a good opportunity for changing some of your unhelpful internal responses. You might also consider seeing a therapist if you find it too difficult to achieve this on your own.

- **Get help from someone to plan your time.** Sometimes it is easier to involve someone else who has a more objective perspective on what is realistic under your circumstances. You may be expecting too much of yourself and it could be good to ask someone else to help you plan your time more realistically.

Chapter 11 in this book on "Problem solving" may also help you think about what you may want to change in your life.

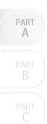

## RECOGNISING YOUR REACTIONS TO STRESS

Once you have identified what may cause stress to you it is important to be aware of your particular reactions to it, as has already been indicated in some of the suggestions, above. However, we are all individuals and therefore the things that may be helpful to a person will differ between people. Research has shown that psychological reactions, such as, whether you think you have control over a situation

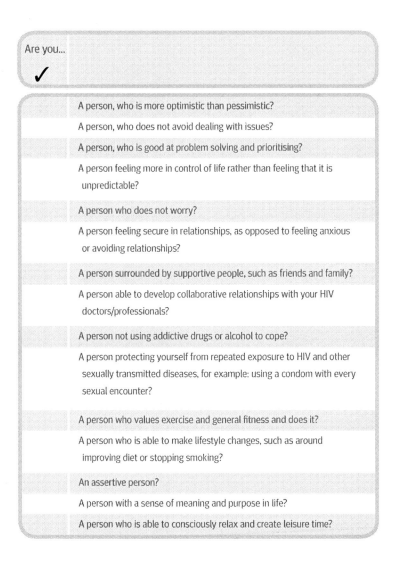

Are you...

✓

A person, who is more optimistic than pessimistic?

A person, who does not avoid dealing with issues?

A person, who is good at problem solving and prioritising?

A person feeling more in control of life rather than feeling that it is unpredictable?

A person who does not worry?

A person feeling secure in relationships, as opposed to feeling anxious or avoiding relationships?

A person surrounded by supportive people, such as friends and family?

A person able to develop collaborative relationships with your HIV doctors/professionals?

A person not using addictive drugs or alcohol to cope?

A person protecting yourself from repeated exposure to HIV and other sexually transmitted diseases, for example: using a condom with every sexual encounter?

A person who values exercise and general fitness and does it?

A person who is able to make lifestyle changes, such as around improving diet or stopping smoking?

An assertive person?

A person with a sense of meaning and purpose in life?

A person who is able to consciously relax and create leisure time?

PART
A

PART
B

PART
C

**Fig. 7** Checklist for Health-related Coping Styles

and your style of coping can influence the course of your illness and how you deal with having it.

In Figure (7) are some reactions that have been associated with some *protection* against disease progression and stress in HIV. In general they are linked to people with a more active, positive coping style. You could use this checklist to see how many factors you rate yourself to have and whether there are some you would like to work on gaining.

Is there anything on this list that you did not tick and that you feel you may like to develop? This will usually involve learning new skills, willingness and effort on your behalf and perhaps additional professional help. We will be offering you the foundation skills in this book that will help in problem solving, dealing with worries and thoughts, mindfulness and relaxation. On the whole the key is developing a balanced lifestyle. Feeling that change is worthwhile and necessary for you, may be your first step.

PART
A

PART
B

PART
C

## WHAT MAKES PEOPLE CHANGE THEIR HEALTH-RELATED BEHAVIOUR?

The *Health Belief Model* (Becker and Rosenstock, 1984) is one of the most popular psychological models used to explain why some people take preventative action, that is to change a health related behaviour in order to prevent unhealthy consequences, and others don't.

According to this model if you want to stop smoking, for example, you will make two main judgements in relation to this:

- How threatening to your health smoking may be.
- To weigh up the pros and cons of taking the action to stop smoking.

Several factors may influence whether you see the first factor of: "perceiving a threat" as applicable to you in relation to smoking, including:

- **How serious the physical and social consequences** are likely to be, if you continue smoking (e.g. developing cancer, lung infections or social rejection). The more serious you see the consequences the more likely you will be to stop.
- **How vulnerable you see yourself to developing physical and social problems** as a result of smoking. The more vulnerable you feel the more likely you are to try and stop (e.g. if you are asthmatic or develop lung cancer).
- **If you are reminded or alerted to the potential health and social problems** resulting from smoking, you may be more likely to stop (e.g. through advertising, your Doctor telling you the health risks and how you can get help to stop).

PART
A

PART
B

PART
C

In relation to the second factor of: "weighing up the pros and cons", you may weigh up whether the benefits you may derive from stopping smoking, such as increased income, better health and relationships, outweigh the barriers you may feel or the personal costs, such as, coping with your feelings of craving or withdrawal if you try and stop.

Why not try and work out now what you may like to change, such as your diet, stopping smoking, drinking alcohol or anything else that you feel would help to improve the health of your life style.

Using the above model go through working out whether you are truly motivated to seek help to change a habit that might be contributing to stress and a less healthy lifestyle in relation to your having HIV? If you identify an area, which you feel you would like to be able to change, but find that you can't find the necessary motivation to make the change, you may like to seek professional help to assist you further with this.

✎ SELF-MONITORING: A CHANCE TO CHECK-IN WITH YOURSELF • *Behavioural change (1) Based on the list of coping styles in Fig. 7 allow yourself some time to work out what coping styles you would like to improve upon? (2) Following this you might like to check-in with yourself to reflect on a particular aspect of your health, which you feel could benefit from improving. What do you need to do differently in order to be able to improve this aspect of your health? It could be very helpful to make some notes about the above in your diary, notebook or on a sheet of paper, so that you can later decide on what might help you to take some of your observations further.*

PART
A

PART
B

PART
C

# RELAXATION – USEFUL PHYSICAL DE-STRESSING TECHNIQUES

Since stress is a part of life, everyone needs to develop methods for "relaxing", or counteracting the physical part of the stress response. Relaxation lowers blood pressure, respiration, and pulse rates, releases muscle tension, and eases emotional strains. There are many relaxation methods and you need to find the ones that suit you. We would like to suggest that you try the following well-known relaxation techniques (Figure 8). If practiced regularly these can be very effective in helping you physically let go of your stresses and deal better with stressful situations. You may also like to read Chapter 9 on mindfulness to help you further with dealing with some of the stressors that life brings you.

## (1) DEEP BREATHING EXERCISES

During stressful situations, breathing becomes shallow and rapid. Taking a slow, deep breath is an effective technique for bringing more oxygen into your body in order to counteract the effects of body tension on your physiology. It can be very useful during a stressful situation, or for maintaining a relaxed state during the day. If you have never done breathing exercises before, you may need to allow yourself some time to practise these, before they will feel easy and pleasant for you to do.

- Inhale through the nose slowly and deeply to the count of eight and hold for four.
- Make sure that the stomach and abdomen expand but the chest does not rise up.
- Exhale through the nose, slowly and completely, also to the count of eight.
- To help quiet the mind, concentrate fully on breathing and counting through each cycle.
- Repeat three times slowly and make a habit of doing the exercise several times each day, even when not feeling stressed.

If you find it very difficult to breathe into your abdomen it can help you to initially lie down and place a heavy book, such as a telephone directory, onto your abdomen. Do the breathing exercise above and gently try to lift the book with each of your in-breaths, counting to eight. Encourage yourself to persevere and stay with it and you will gain a pleasant sense of mastery!

PART
A

PART
B

PART
C

**Fig. 8** Two Methods of Relaxation (cont. over page)

## (2) PROGRESSIVE MUSCULAR RELAXATION

Muscle relaxation techniques can be combined with deep breathing, are simple to learn and very useful for teaching you to recognise body tension and to help getting you to sleep. Practice makes this exercise much more effective and produces relaxation much more rapidly in the day as you learn to recognise the difference between tension and relaxation in all the major muscle groups and can then check this out regularly in the course of the day. Sometimes, to help you learn this form of relaxation it could be helpful to see a health professional, such as a Clinical Psychologist, who is trained to teach this. This form of relaxation is also sometimes taught as part of Yoga or Meditation Classes, which it could be helpful for you to attend.

PART A

PART B

PART C

- After lying down in a comfortable position without crossing your limbs, concentrate on each part of your body.
- Maintain a slow, deep breathing pattern throughout this exercise.
- Tense each muscle as tightly as possible for a count of five as you breathe in and then release it completely as you breathe out slowly.
- Experience the muscle as totally relaxed and lead-heavy.
- Begin with the toes and progress upward through your body to focus on all the muscle groups in the body.
- Be sure to include the feet, calves, knees, thighs, lower back, belly, chest, mid- and upper back, fingers, hands, forearms, upper arms, shoulders, neck, chin area, mouth, cheeks, eyes, forehead, ears and scalp area.
- Once the external review is complete, imagine tensing and releasing internal muscles.
- Lie back and enjoy feeling completely relaxed for as long as you want.

# CONCLUSION

This chapter has focussed on stress, its effects and ways to help you manage stress. There are many types of stress associated with HIV and some of them are unpredictable, but being more aware of your role in at least reducing the effects of some of the stressors, especially the self-created ones, will make a difference.

The more aware you are of the obstacles, the more choices you will have in your actions and therefore you are more able to make a plan that works around change. Especially, allow yourself to recognize some old habits or patterns, which you may always have engaged in, but that now on reflection actually, may no longer work for you because they are not helpful to your current situation. Allow yourself to take this period in your life as an opportunity for internal change. You may find that despite the challenges that living with HIV presents, you can actually achieve greater internal freedom if you allow yourself to make some of the changes that give you greater choice and enhance the health of your lifestyle. However, allow yourself to be patient and kind to yourself and remember that most things take time to turn around. Give yourself credit for those steps that you have already undertaken making some of these changes. It can be done!

PART
A

PART
B

PART
C

# Negotiating HIV Treatment, Healthcare & Social Care

# INTRODUCTION

We know that being HIV positive can be extremely challenging. Being involved in your own medical treatment, and getting help from your healthcare centre when needed, can improve your quality of life, coping skills and help you live longer.

Your healthcare centre is likely to offer lots of services provided by different health professionals (e.g. dieticians, clinical psychologists, nurses), as well as, medical care. There are also lots of services and support available from community-based organisations like the 'Elton John Foundation', 'Body and Soul' and 'The Terence Higgins' Trust' found in London. This means that you will potentially have access to a very large support networks with HIV. Getting to grips with these is important so that you can feel more in control of your health monitoring and treatments, and have people you can rely on at different points in the course of your condition. You may well at times have felt isolated and alone living with HIV. This is completely understandable given the stigma associated with HIV and around disclosure. The idea of getting more involved with people may be frightening, but our experience has been that it can really help people to feel better in the long run.

PART A

PART B

PART C

This chapter attempts to help you think about what your network is and how best to use it for the benefit of your health. It will focus on your relationship with important members of your network: your HIV Medical Doctor and how you can feel more in control of negotiating HIV treatment, and, also, how you can access psychological help and other support organisations.

# WHAT IS YOUR CURRENT NETWORK OF CARE?

It is very important that you are fully aware of all the services and people that you may be linked into and that you know what further support might be on offer. This helps you to feel more in control of your care and able to ask for additional support when you may need it and feel confident in what you are receiving.

You may find it helpful to use Figure (9), to try and map out the people and services you currently rely on. Put yourself in the centre and the services around you. These could include partners, relatives, community groups, the Church or other spiritual support groups, HIV drop-in centres, clinics, G.P, HIV wards, physiotherapists, dieticians, clinical psychologists, psychotherapists, social workers, benefits advisers, and so on.

PART
A

PART
B

PART
C

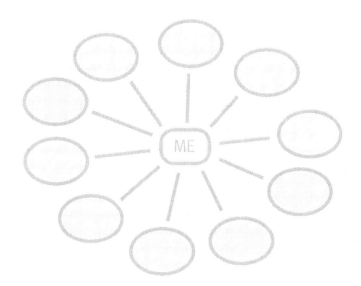

Fig. 9 My HIV network

Did you manage to fill out many of the circles or were there many empty gaps? You may find yourself isolated. This may be particularly difficult if you are newly diagnosed and are worried about being judged by others, if you tell them about having HIV when you ask for help.

Is this the case for you? Is it excluding you from support you might need, such as someone to talk to about your worries or practical aspects of having HIV? We shall think about how to face fears of stigma in the next chapter. Becoming part of a network of care and support and feeling more able to negotiate the resources that could be supportive to you, will help you cope better with having HIV in the long run.

On the other hand you may find yourself running out of circles to fill as you have a very large social and care network. If this is the case, is it clear to you, who is co-ordinating your care (e.g. usually a doctor, social worker or nurse)? Is it clear in your mind, who you would call on for what and how to contact them? Are you happy with the resources that are currently provided for you?

In both instances, above, after having thought about the services, resources and support available to you a little more closely, you may like to take some steps to build a greater or better coordinated supportive network, such as, gathering more information or clarifying the different roles that the people supporting you currently take or discussing further what is available and what your needs are with your treatment centre.

PART
A

PART
B

PART
C

# DIFFERENT STYLES OF HELP-SEEKING

The two cases, below, illustrate the importance of good support and communication with your care network in order for you to be able to cope well with your condition.

Alice *is aged 37 and has been HIV positive for two years. When she visits the hospital for her blood test for Viral Load and CD4 Counts, she becomes fearful shortly before the date, because she is afraid of possible bad news. Lately, she has been worrying about a skin rash, which she fears could mean that she might be getting ill due to her HIV and she also worries about bumping into someone she might know in the hospital. She has not disclosed her HIV status to anyone and feels very isolated, as she has no one to talk her worries through with. When at the hospital, Alice is filled with fear because she sees hospitals as places where people go when they are ill. When she is with her doctor, she doesn't say much or ask any questions, but is relieved when the doctor says that her counts are good and she does not need any medication. After leaving the hospital she returns home relieved if she did not bump into anyone she knew. However, she feels very alone with and isolated in her experience.*

Sam *is aged 24 and has also been HIV positive for two years. When he visits the hospital for his blood test for Viral Load and CD4 Counts, he does so in a relatively calm manner.*
*He has disclosed his HIV status to some close friends and has discussed his feelings with them about being HIV positive. When at the hospital, Sam chats with the staff. He is feeling supported and open about being HIV positive. In his consultation with his doctor, he explains the concerns he has about the benefits he needs and his HIV symptoms. As a result of this discussion, Sam receives a referral to a service, which can help him with his benefits and some new medication to treat the symptoms, Sam has been concerned with. Subsequently, Sam leaves the hospital feeling supported and cared for.*

In Chapter 4 we shall be looking at how to overcome the barriers of shame, stigma, the difficulty in accepting the diagnosis and the very common feelings of isolation in relation to having HIV. All the above may affect your ability to engage with others who could support you and therefore limit the range of support available to you. Alice has many adjustment concerns that she will feel left with and frightened about if she does not find ways of overcoming some of her fears and get help for her concerns surrounding the issues connected to having HIV.

Sam, on the other hand, is more able to draw on the support from the relationships within his care network and seems to be more able to share his concerns relating to issues of adjusting to the virus. As a result, he feels less anxious, less isolated and is able to cope better. Central to this process is his social network, especially the people who can support him in a practical and emotional way and encourage his active participation in his care. We shall now guide you in thinking through some of the issues that might be helpful in improving matters, in relation to the care and support networks around you, starting with your relationship to your HIV doctor.

PART
A

PART
B

PART
C

# GETTING THE BEST OUT OF
# YOUR MEDICAL DOCTOR

You have probably seen quite a lot of doctors since you were first diagnosed HIV positive (and many other health professionals) and may have found that you felt more comfortable with some rather than others. This is to be expected – each professional will have his or her particular ways of interacting. Depending on personality, background experience and other factors, some professionals will find it easier to relate to some people, but not others. Therefore, you will feel more comfortable with some but not other professionals. However, we know from research that it is very important that you do feel very comfortable with your doctor. Your relationship with your doctor is very important and when it feels right, it helps you play an active role in negotiating and planning your HIV treatment. The better your relationship or "alliance" with your doctor, the more likely you are to be happy with the care you receive, as you will feel actively included in shaping this. You will also feel less distress about what is happening in your illness and be more likely to collaborate with the treatment plans made for you, because you will understand these, as you would have been actively involved.

Researchers have spent a lot of time looking at relationships between doctors and patients and they discovered the things that made patients happier when talking to their doctor and more satisfied with the outcome of their visit. These were:

- The doctor being friendly rather than businesslike
- The doctor being seen as understanding their patients' concerns
- Patients' expectations about their treatments were being met
- The doctor being perceived as a good communicator
- Appropriate and understandable provision of information

In addition they found that patients:

- often did not understand the words that were used by the doctor
- often had their own ideas about illnesses and treatments, and that these differed from the accepted ideas of the doctor
- were reluctant to ask for more information even when they would very much have liked to

- often forgot a great deal of what they were told,
  especially, if they had a low level of medical knowledge
  and experienced some level of anxiety
- remembered the first piece of information given best
  and also information that was simplified, categorised,
  repeated, and made specific by the doctor
- experienced telephoned and mailed reminders helpful
  and also the provision of written back-up material

Our experience has been that people often feel reluctant to talk to their doctor about issues and concerns because they think that the doctor or the clinic is too busy and they feel bad about taking up more of their time. While clinics are often busy places, most doctors will be happy to try and address issues that you bring up. Even when they are busy, considering the above factors, it is important that you try and make your doctor aware of any concerns or new issues that have arisen for you. The more your doctor understands you and your concerns, the more likely you are to receive the help that you actually need. It is also true that your doctor may not always have time to check everything with you on every visit. Your doctor will therefore be relying on you to some extent to raise any new concerns or issues that have arisen! This makes it important for you to try and prepare for your visit so that you are able to discuss what you want with your doctor.

The above information might have helped you to realize how important it is for you to prepare for the visits to your doctor, irrespective of how anxious you may feel. You may also have started to recognize that you have choices in your relationship with your doctor. Here is a tip, which might be useful. In general, it can help for you to plan your visit by writing lists of questions relating to your care and

PART
A

PART
B

PART
C

bringing them to an appointment. It could be useful to have a place in your home where you keep a notebook and whenever you think of a concern in relation to your symptoms or any issues relating to your medical care, you could make a note of this. Before your next visit to your doctor, you may like to go through the things you have noted down and highlight those, which are still relevant for you. You could then take this with you on your next visit and share this with your doctor. This may enable you to have a more satisfying two-way conversation with your doctor, which, in turn, will usually create a good foundation for your shared care.

Obviously, as in other areas of your life it is not always possible to get on with everyone. So if, despite some attempts from your side to build a good relationship with your doctor, you still do not feel comfortable enough with your doctor to raise the things, which you feel would be important for you to share, it is perfectly within your right to change your doctor. Sometimes, this may be the best solution, especially if you have heard or even might know of another doctor, who you feel you could have a better relationship with. This may enable you to establish a more actively engaged relationship with your new doctor right from the beginning.

Below, is an example to help you think through some of the issues that Mark was facing with his doctor, which are not uncommon.

*Mark found that his sessions with his doctor were quite short so the conversation revolved mainly around his viral load and CD4 blood count, which were responding well to the drugs he was taking. However Mark was experiencing difficult side effects such as nausea, lipodystrophy (abnormal body fat redistribution) and depression, which he found difficult to talk about, because it brought up some distressing emotions in him when he thought about this. When he took the courage to raise his concerns he felt they were minimised by his doctor, as his focus was on how well his immunity was. The doctor encouraged him to persevere with the medication, which seemed to work for him with other clients.*

How helpful do you find Mark's relationship with his doctor? What do you suspect would make Mark more satisfied with his medical consultations? How could he prepare for his next meeting with his doctor? What questions should Mark ask his doctor the next time he has an appointment? After allowing yourself to go through some of the concerns Mark has with his doctor, you might like to write down a similar scenario of your own experiences with your doctor. This may enable you to examine more objectively, whether there are any things, which you feel need to be improved or changed concerning the relationship with your doctor.

PART
A

PART
B

PART
C

# COPING WITH HIV MEDICATION

Starting combination therapies will be an important moment and transition in your life and is likely to raise many hopes and fears. Your psychological and emotional reactions to taking combination therapies are equally important to consider along with the physical demands of taking the pills.

We would like to suggest therefore that it is well worth setting some time aside to think carefully about how you feel about starting combination therapies? It could be helpful for you to consider the following three questions:

* (1) What do the drugs mean to you and your life, as you currently see it?
* (2) What are your hopes connected to taking these drugs?
* (3) What are your current fears?

Your hopes connected to the combination therapies may include staying well and healthy. Some of your fears may include having your life always dictated by the pills rather than remaining your own boss over your life. Another concern might be that each time you take the drugs you are being reminded that you are HIV positive. You may also not like the idea of having to take constant chemicals into your body, especially, if so far, you have tried to lead a relatively natural life style. You may also be concerned about some of the possible side effects of taking these drugs. These or other reactions are completely understandable given how life changing the start of combination therapies can be. It is important to share your concerns with your doctor and other health professionals in your treatment centre. If these are not adequately addressed you may find that you feel too anxious or might become depressed. This could then get in the way of you starting or continuing with the combination therapies, even though they would be helpful for you.

Collaboration with your doctor around regular checkups, which might include viral load testing and $CD_4$ blood count to check on your immune status and decisions about treatment and medication follow-up, will play a central role in your relationship with your doctor and other health professionals. It is quite natural that you will have many doubts and questions around HIV and its treatment. Correct and accurate information is usually available from your doctor and the HIV unit you are supported by. Some of the most important decisions around having HIV will concern the timing of when to start combination therapies and which ones to take. Usually, doctors recommend starting medication if you are unwell, or when you feel well, but have between 200-350 CD4 cells per cubic millimetre (mm³) in your blood. There are many drugs now available and up-to-date information about these is available from reliable sources, such as the National AIDS Manual (www.aidsmap.com). Considerations of side effects, drug interactions, how often to take the pills, the dosage of pills, lifestyle and other issues, such as pregnancy, are often considered in the final choice of drugs that will be the right ones for you.

Obviously, once you and your doctor have decided that it would be helpful to start combination therapy, it will be important that you take the drugs, in the way that is recommended for the specific drugs that have been identified for you. This is called adherence to taking drugs. There are many reasons why people may not adhere to taking the drugs, in the way in which they have been prescribed. For example, they may forget to take their drugs regularly, or they may not take the right dosage or they may not take them continuously, because they feel that they are starting to feel better again.

Unfortunately, with combination therapy it is very important that the drugs are taken as prescribed. It can have negative consequences on the way in which HIV progresses, if people don't take their drugs at the right time continuously as prescribed in the medication packet. It has been found that there are *two significant factors*, which contribute to people's poor adherence with their drug therapy. The *first* of these is related to your understanding of the pros and cons of your drug treatment and the *second* is related to misplaced beliefs about the relative risks and benefits of treatment. Correct information upon which to base your decisions and adequate support in helping you

PART
A

PART
B

PART
C

to make them are therefore essential. It is very important for you to find the courage to ask questions and to find out as much information about the drugs that you are taking as you need. This will help you to take them regularly and in the right dosage.

Below, is a list of potential problems that might face you when wanting to take your suggested drugs. As you go through the list, if you identify any that feel relevant to your decisions around drug treatment, it might be very helpful to discuss them with your health care team or doctor. If you do decide to take drugs and are prescribed drugs it is important to follow the medical advice on dosages and duration of the drug taking. This is, because not doing so, could result in a number of adverse consequences for you.

These include:

- Drug resistance, which is when the drugs that used to attack the HIV virus, don't have any effect anymore, because the virus has changed its structure
- Drug rebound effects, which result in an increase in symptoms after a drug has been stopped
- Further illness

It is also important that you report any side effects, which are unwanted symptoms caused by using a particular medicine, rather than a disease, such as, for example, diarrhoea, to your doctor or health care team. There may be ways of dealing with them or you may require a change in medication. However, you need the help of an HIV specialist, who has knowledge of the range of medication available to help you with this.

# POTENTIAL BARRIERS TO TAKING HIV MEDICATION

Figure (10) shows a variety of barriers to taking medication. Are any of the following an issue for you?

---

### PHYSICAL TREATMENT FACTORS

- Number of tablets you have to take
- Size of the tablets that have been prescribed
- Other characteristics of the tablets, such as taste or smell
- Inadequate labelling or unsuitable containers or seals on the packaging of the tablets
- Complexity of the drug taking regimen, such as the frequency and timing being too complicated
- Drug taking regimen that interferes with your lifestyle, such as bedtime or social activities
- Intolerability or toxicity of the drugs, leading to side-effects
- Multiple medications, making them difficult to swallow or to plan or to tolerate
- Long duration of treatment
- Expense of either some of the drugs or the special diet you need to accompany your therapy
- Side-effects (i.e. diarrhoea, headaches, feeling sick, rashes, lipodystrophy, neuropathy)

---

PART
A

PART
B

PART
C

**Fig. 10** Barriers to Treatment (cont. over page)

## PERSONAL PRACTICAL/PHYSICAL CHARACTERISTICS

* Extremes of age, for example, you may be so young, that it might not make sense to you to start to take drugs regularly at your age
* Homeless/poor living conditions with nowhere to store the drugs, or other problems
* Difficulty in attending the clinic, such as due to distance or lack of childcare facilities
* Difficulty in disclosing HIV status to companions, work colleagues, family or friends
* Poor social support and sense of isolation, may make it hard to motivate yourself to take drugs
* Severity of your illness. If you are very ill or feel confused this may be a problem
* Significant alcohol or recreational use of other drugs may interfere with the prescribed drugs
* Sensory disabilities (e.g. blind) may make it difficult to adhere to the instructions
* Language, for example, difficulty reading the instructions or communicating the concerns about the drug regimen or side effects

## PERSONAL PSYCHOLOGICAL/MOTIVATIONAL CHARACTERISTICS

* Aversion to taking any drugs
* Concerns about taking a specific drug
* Beliefs about the severity of the disease, such as failure to see the need for treatment because it is hard to see the disease as life threatening

- Negative expectations of the likely outcome of therapy, such as, feeling that the drugs may not be able to help
- Dissatisfaction with the treatment that has been received so far
- Apathy or fatalism about having HIV, such as, feeling there is no point anyway
- Emotional problems, including depression
- Life events that cause emotional turmoil, such as relationship breakdown
- Lack of understanding of the importance of adherence or poor knowledge of the required treatment regimen
- Poor memory (forgetting medication) or confusion or dementia
- Cultural beliefs or particular rituals that interfere with the taking of conventional medicines
- Belief that regular or long-term medication is unnecessary
- Embarrassment or stigma associated with having to use medication
- Concerns about the adverse effects of taking the medication

PART
A

PART
B

PART
C

## PERSONAL-PRACTITIONER INTERACTION

- Feeling that your doctor or other health professionals in the team have a negative attitude to the social group you are part of
- Inadequate communication, such as lack of advice, inconsistent or conflicting information
- Failure of your doctor or other health professionals to elicit feedback about your problems or difficulties with the recommended therapy
- Inadequate follow up or monitoring of your medical needs
- Lack of continuity of care, such as due to changes in healthcare

professionals, lack of resources or other factors

• Dissatisfaction with your doctor or other professional healthcare support, such as unsatisfactory communication; contact not frequent enough; too frequent changes in healthcare staff, etc.

If you have identified any of the factors listed, above, to be barriers for you, it might be helpful for you to write these down. Some of the problems listed can be overcome by following practical measures that you may also wish to discuss with your health care professional or doctor. It is important that you feel able and willing to follow the advice that is given to you by your doctor or healthcare team. Therefore, it is important that you do not feel rushed into any decisions that may later lead to poor adherence to your treatment. You could take the list of those factors that you consider to be obstacles for you to your doctor or another health care professional and explore them together.

PART A

PART B

PART C

## IMPORTANCE OF GOOD ADHERENCE

The terms 'adherence' and 'compliance' are used interchangeably but roughly mean the same thing. They refer to the extent to which a person adequately follows the prescription for the medicine. As we have previously outlined, in order for your drugs to have the desired effect of slowing down the HIV progress, a very good adherence or compliance rate is necessary. Over 95% adherence (taking your drugs 95% absolutely correctly in terms of timing and dosage) is vital to the success of HIV antiretrovirals. Any factor that may interfere with your adherence to regular drug taking needs to be addressed. As outlined, above, these might include pill burden or having too many pills to take, the dosing frequency, adverse side effects, factors relating to mood and life circumstances.

The following medication "compliance aids" could help you to overcome some of the practical problems you may have with taking the drugs:

- Alarm watches or message pagers to remind you of the right time to take your drugs
- Daily or weekly pill boxes with compartments for each dose time
- Medication record cards
- Stickers for drug bottles or cartons with boxes for dates and times to check off when the doses have been taken

PART
A

PART
B

PART
C

You can usually get help in discussing what might support you in your efforts to take your medication regularly and reliably or your problems with taking drugs at your HIV centre. There are often pharmacists or nurses you can address these issues with in addition to your own doctor. They can help you to obtain specific pillboxes, or to make a plan, or help you to talk to your doctor about the support you need in order to be able to successfully manage your adherence.

# SIDE-EFFECTS

In our experience most people living with HIV who start medication are concerned about side-effects. This is completely understandable given that at best they can be a real nuisance and, at worst, can make you feel very unwell. That is why for many people who need to start medication the issue of side-effects is an important one. You may well know of other HIV positive people who started medication and experience quite bad side-effects. This will understandably make you wonder whether the same could happen to you. In talking about side-effects with you, we would like to inform rather than alarm, although we realise it is entirely natural for you to have concerns about them.

It is important that you are aware of any changes in your body that are occurring as a result of being HIV positive. These may be signs of illness or health. Also, frequently, people experience side effects due to the HIV drug treatments, which can affect their quality of life significantly. If you are noticing any changes, either physical or psychological, in conjunction with the taking of your medication, informing your doctor will be very important. The sooner you report any of these changes the quicker can appropriate management and advice be provided for you. Alternative therapies and other medications can also sometimes help to control some of the side effects, but it is very important that you always consult your doctor to avoid bad drug interactions from occurring.

Some of the sensations or physical feelings you are experiencing may not be side-effects, but could be symptoms in their own right. They could be a sign of other illnesses such as chest infections. Therefore it is very important that you still report them as soon as you notice them, so that appropriate help can be provided for you.

You may like to use the side-effect diary in Figure 11 (p.86) to record any changes in your health that could be related to the side effects of taking drugs. We have given an example of how you could use it. You may or may not have any side effects, but it is important to observe and record and disclose any that do occur. There are many advantages to recording information in this way. For instance, it could provide your doctor with useful information about how much side-effects affect you, or help you to monitor improvements to side-effects you may be experiencing. Below, are some common side-effects. They may seem quite overwhelming to you upon first reading them, as there are quite a few. Please remember that in order to provide you with as much information as possible, we have included the most common side-effects. This does not mean that you will get all of them! We know from experience that some people are lucky and experience very few side-effects, while others can feel very unwell, because of the side-effects of treatment. Unfortunately there is no easy way to predict what will happen to you, so this understandably could make you feel nervous when you start or change medication.

Common Side-Effects are:

(1) Tingling in your hands or feet

(2) Pain in your hands or feet

(3) Nausea or vomiting

(4) Headache

(5) Feeling tired

(6) Changes to your eyesight or vision

(7) Dry skin

(8) Rash

(9) Diarrhoea

(10) Stomach pains

(11) Hair loss

(12) Body shape changes

(13) Weight gain or weight loss

(14) Changes in your taste or appetite

PART
A

PART
B

PART
C

(15) Sexual problems

(16) Sleep disturbance

(17) Vivid dreaming

(18) Feeling anxious or nervous

(19) Mood swings or feeling depressed

(20) Any other symptoms you have noticed:

| SIDE-EFFECT SYMPTOM | FREQUENCY How often do the symptoms occur? | DURATION How long do the symptoms last? | SEVERITY Scale: 1 = very mild 10 = very bad | AFFECTED AREA OF LIFE Describe |
|---|---|---|---|---|
| diarrhoea | 5 times a day | 5 mins | 6 | socialising |
| | | | | |
| | | | | |
| | | | | |
| | | | | |
| | | | | |
| | | | | |

Fig. 11 Side-effect diary

**SELF-MONITORING: A CHANCE TO CHECK-IN WITH YOURSELF** • *Your doctor and your medication* (1) *Allow yourself some time to think about your medical doctor and your relationship with him/her at the moment. What are the areas that work well and what are the areas, where there could be improvement? (2) You might like to check-in with yourself to reflect on the issues that you are facing right now with your medication. How is your adherence? Do you experience any side effects? Also if you are not on any medication are there any worries you have about taking this in the future? It could be very helpful to make some notes about the above in your diary, notebook or on a sheet of paper, so that you can later decide on what might help you to take some of your observations further.*

PART
A

PART
B

PART
C

# WHEN IN-PATIENT CARE IS NEEDED

You may already have spent some time in hospital feeling unwell, because of your HIV. It is also possible that you may have been unwell in hospital for other reasons, perhaps as a child, for instance or because of an accident. Nearly all of us though will have visited a hospital either to see friends or family or as an outpatient. Each one of us has their own experiences and memories of hospitals that influence our feelings and expectations about them. For some of you it may just be a memory of a strong and unusual smell, for others happy memories of a birth of a child or sibling, whilst some of you may have sad memories of losing someone close to you in hospital.

Due to the existence and continuous progress of combination drug treatments, in-patient care for complications of HIV is less frequent.

However, despite a much more hopeful outlook in the management of HIV, there may nevertheless be times when you are admitted to hospital with HIV-related conditions, which require in-patient treatment. This would, for example, be the case if you suffered from pneumonia, or it might apply in order to help stabilise the medication side-effects, and, obviously, when there are terminal conditions. The last is fortunately rare these days and usually associated with people who present late in their condition when their immune system is already considerably jeopardised or when severe resistance to the medication has developed as a result of patchy adherence or length of treatment and complications.

Again in talking with you about the issues of inpatient care, we hope to inform rather than alarm you. We realise though that it is entirely natural to have some fears about being in hospital. What we would like to suggest to you is that having some information about staying in hospital and spending a bit of time thinking about in advance, could help reduce some of the concerns and fears you may have. For example, hospital wards are unfamiliar places, and you may find that having with you a few familiar items from home, like photographs of people close to you, may help you to feel a bit more comfortable.

Usually going into hospital is a difficult time as you may be trying to:

- Make sense of your physical symptoms and care and what this will mean for you and your close ones. This can relate to practical matters, such as changes to your working life and childcare, but it can also affect you emotionally and physically, such as coming to terms with disability, illness or grief. Some hospitals have multi-faith chaplainries, who will come and talk to you while you are an inpatient. You may want to consider if this would be helpful for you.
- Get used to an unfamiliar place with unfamiliar routines. Lights often

go out late or you may be woken early; there will be different noises to relate to and, on the whole, you will experience far less privacy.

- Keep yourself occupied and in touch with loved ones with fewer of your usual props, such as your mobile phone and household things. You are advised not to bring in valuables, have few of your own clothes to wear, and may not have the same access to books, games, T.V. and other things that may have kept you occupied at home. Usually there is access to a pay phone at the bedside and a television. However, this may be shared with others.
- Understand the different roles of staff in hospital, as it may be difficult to know who is responsible for which part of your care and to whom you should talk if you have any questions or concerns.

The roles of hospital staff can include the following:

- *Consultant*, who will have the overall responsibility for your medical care.
- *Ward Manager* (or Senior Sister, Matron), who is responsible for the day to day running of the ward who will allocate nurses to your nursing care.
- *Physiotherapist*, who will be involved in your care if you are experiencing difficulty with walking or moving, or breathing.
- *Occupational Therapist*, who may be asked to assess what daily living tasks you are able to carry out, such as preparing meals or going to the toilet or preparing meals or drinks. They may recommend or provide aids or adaptations to enable you to undertake these tasks. Sometimes they may accompany you on a visit home before you are discharged to see if you could cope on your own with daily living tasks and whether you need any equipment to help reduce risks.

PART
A

PART
B

PART
C

- *Hospital Social Worker,* who would be responsible for coordinating an assessment of your support needs once you leave hospital. They may arrange for these services for when you leave hospital.
- *Dietician,* who is trained to assess your dietary requirements and how nutrition can best be taken and provided. For example, if a person is unable to swallow fluid or food as assessed by a speech and language therapist the nutritionist can plan and monitor any equipment that would help to overcome this difficulty.

PART
A

PART
B

PART
C

If you have developed a good collaborative relationship with your doctor and healthcare team this will considerably help you through the experience of being an in-patient, should the need for this arise. In a supportive and collaborative healthcare environment, you will be able to negotiate your needs and express your concerns with more ease. In-patient units can appear strange, busy and clinical places at the best of times. Sometimes, this can make you feel less able to ask questions that you may feel you need answered, such as what will happen to you in a procedure, or be updated on your treatment plan.

Whilst being in hospital you have the right to expect high standards of treatment and care, which includes:

- The right to be involved in all decisions about your treatment and be kept informed
- The right to name any relative or friend to be informed about your condition
- The right to see your medical records
- The right to be treated with dignity and have your religious and cultural beliefs respected
- The right to have your nutritional needs upheld and assessed

If you are in the unfortunate position of feeling unhappy with your treatment, you should raise your concerns with the hospital staff. This can be done by firstly, talking things through with the ward sister and then taking matters to the manager or your consultant. Tell them what you are unhappy with and what you would like to see improved. If you feel you need help with this in the U.K., your local Patient Advice and Liaison Service (PALS), which is found in all hospitals, should be able to help you try and resolve the issue you may be dissatisfied with. Also, your named friend or relative, could play an active role in helping you sort things out so that you feel more content and satisfied with your treatment in hospital or the hospital environment.

PART
A

# DYING AND HIV

PART
B

PART
C

HIV will always be associated with death and dying. Perhaps one of the first things you thought about when you were diagnosed or heard about someone having HIV is that theirs or your life will be shorter. As you have progressed in your illness over some time or if you presented late with a weakened immune system, as a result of having contracted HIV, you might think death is imminent. This may lead you to go through a process of coming to terms with the possibility of death. For most people this is an extremely difficult emotional stage and you, as well as, those close to this process may feel considerably affected.

There is no easy way of dealing with the possibility of your own death or the death of others that are close to you. Coming to terms and understanding death is a very individual process and for most people it brings up many differing emotions and requires time. There are also no easy ways of helping you to come to terms with the possibility of your own death or the death of a person dear to you. It is a process that can't be learnt abstractly or taken from text books, nor can other people advice you how it should be done. It requires going through it and allowing yourself to stay as fully connected to the process as you can tolerate. This includes allowing yourself all the emotions and bodily feelings that may come up for you during this process. It can be extremely helpful to have the support and nurturing of some close friends or healthcare professionals who you trust, while you are going through this process. However, this may also be difficult for you while you are going through this phase, as it may connect you with feelings of wanting to disengage with others rather than staying connected. Sometimes, the feelings of connection can make the pain associated with the possibility of your own death even stronger.

Many people, when facing the possibility of their own death or the death of a person close to them go through several stages. Although, there is no way in which this process can be made easy or carried by others, it can be helpful for you to have some understanding of the stages, which you might be going through. While not being able to relieve you of your process, it might provide you with some validation and understanding that you are not alone in experiencing some of these feelings or going through these stages. They are normal and necessary, despite being difficult and painful. Professor Elizabeth Kübler-Ross (1969), probably one of the most well-known psychologists working in this area, has observed five stages, which most people follow through in their process of coming to terms with dying and death. She noted that hope can thread its way throughout the sequence and that the stages do not necessarily have to follow in exact order. Although it may be very difficult for you to read, it could help you in your understanding of your own process of coming to terms with dying and death.

Grief is a normal, healthy response to loss, although it can feel overwhelming, upsetting and confusing. As you face the prospect of dying, you may have different feelings at different times. These feelings can relate to:

* Shock
* Denial
* Anger
* Guilt
* Sadness
* Acceptance

You may find yourself going back and forth from one feeling to another. For example, right when it seems that you're starting to accept that you are dying, you may find yourself feeling sad.

In the first hours or days of finding out that you have a fatal illness, you may feel shocked, numb, confused and stunned. You may think and act as though it isn't true, but be preoccupied and dazed at the same time. The evidence cannot quite sink in.

As your shock wears off reality may start to sink in. You may begin to realize that your life may end. At this stage people can find themselves feeling let down and angry. If you have these feelings they would be entirely normal and understandable. Your anger may shift from one target to another and you may find yourself snapping at loved ones, your doctor, or even at God for the unfairness of the situation. At times your anger may feel more like actual rage, at other times you may experience feelings of bitterness and resentment.

You may find yourself working through some of the anger and denial and after this, you may become more thoughtful and willing to

PART
A

PART
B

PART
C

make a deal with fate, yourself or God. It is normal to try and pretend things are like they used to be and a measure of hope and belief in your abilities may have been reawakened inside you.

If your condition worsens and you become weaker, more tired and less able to function, you may become quite vulnerable to depression. This can be a very difficult time, indeed - perhaps the worst, as you may be faced with fear of death. However, this dread is usually replaced soon after by acceptance of the situation and you may become aware of a tremendous calm inside you as this starts to happen. You may begin to realise that dying is a process that everyone will have to undertake as part of their lifetime, at some stage. Ultimately, irrespective of the circumstances and the differing situations people are in, dying is a part of living that each person has to face. This process cannot be taken on and done by others for you or indeed, for anybody else in this world. Therefore, you may feel tremendously alone, for dying is ultimately a process that every person has to undergo alone. Others may comfort, be there for you and support you, but they cannot go through this process for you. Indeed, they, in their own time shall have to go through that very same process for themselves on their own. The process of dying, whatever the circumstances, poses challenges to every human being. It might require you to accomplish some or most of the following tasks:

- Psychological tasks can include finding meaning in death and suffering in order to help you gain more understanding of yourself and the process you are going through. It may lift your fear and you may learn to accept what is happening to you.
- Social tasks can include telling people you care about your situation, dealing with their reactions and coming to terms

with the ending of your attachments to others in this world.

- Physical tasks can include coming to terms with the loss of physical functioning, such as restricted activity, loss of energy, changes in your body image, and dealing with pain or disability. Writing of a "living will" where you work out your terminal care treatment wishes and let all those involved in your care know about these (for example, stopping treatment when you are on a ventilator, if there is little chance of recovery). This can ease some of your anxieties and give you and those close to you comfort, as they understand your wishes.

- Practical tasks can include the writing of wills, stating your funeral wishes, tidying your financial affairs, disposing of unwanted material things and withdrawing from your responsibilities in life, such as work.

- Spiritual tasks can include finding and affirming meaning of what is happening to you in religious or spiritual terms, having a sense of connectedness, transcendence and hope.

PART
A

PART
B

PART
C

Naturally, facing your own death is likely to be extremely difficult. You may find that those around you find it hard to talk about it with you. This could be because they fear it could upset you. They may also be finding it hard to deal with their own feelings about your death, such as being able to accept that you are dying. While these are understandable reactions, these may be very difficult and hard for you to cope with. It is also possible that others stop talking to you about normal things in life, like going out and having a good time, because they fear this could be insensitive and upsetting to you. At this stage it is important that you allow yourself to be as honest as you can with yourself and with others. You may find that it is important for you to say to others what you would find helpful and not helpful during this time. For example, saying that you would still like to hear about what is going on in their lives, if this is what would help you. It may feel really important to you that you are included, rather than kept out, of their lives.

Although, dying and death are natural processes, which we all have to face, in Western society we have lost connection to these. Of course, dying and death happens all throughout the world many times every day, however, in our Western culture it is kept away from people's everyday experiences. It feels to many of us as if it happens outside normal, daily life. We may watch it on a cinema screen, on television or see and read about it in the newspapers. However, we are rarely part of it in our daily lives, apart from our experience of the deaths of our direct relatives, such as parents, siblings or partners. If death does happen, our society is organized in a way that deals with it very efficiently, almost in a parallel world, without impacting too much on other people's lives. Therefore, many of us have not come across death very often and when we have to face our own death it can feel like a very lonely experience. We may feel quite isolated, abandoned and left alone with it.

If you are able to and when you sense that you might soon be approaching the stage in your illness where your own death feels a real possibility to you, it might be helpful to visualize in your mind how you would like your own death to be. Who would be the people that you would like most around you during the last stages in your life? How would you like the environment in which you die to be? How would you like the professionals to treat and interact with you at this stage? What else would be important for you in order to enable you a peaceful passage and transition from this life? It might feel difficult for you to do this exercise, because you are not quite ready to face the possibility of your own death, yet. However, it could be helpful if you allowed yourself to overcome your fear of doing this exercise at a stage in your life, where you still have much control over expressing your desires and needs. You would then be able to share your vision with those people who you trust most and feel closest to and together you could work out which aspects of this vision, you would like them to help you realize. You might find, if you are able to share and express your own wishes in this way that you may approach your death in a peaceful and calm state and this stage of final change and transition may feel more like a natural, inevitable part of your life.

# ACCESSING A PROFESSIONAL
# FOR MENTAL HEALTH CONCERNS

PART
A

PART
B

PART
C

There may be times when you feel you may like to discuss what you are thinking and feeling in relation to your illness in more depth in a confidential and safe environment away from your home and your usual relationships. It is common as you are going through your illness to feel anxious, frightened and depressed. You may also feel it could be helpful to have support during the times when you have to make difficult adjustments and decisions around your illness, such as, taking time off work; disclosing your HIV status; exploring which people are helpful people and potentially good friends to have around or when to start taking combination drugs and others.

Talking therapies involve talking and listening. Most of us find it helpful to talk to somebody, who listens and accepts us, especially when we are going through a bad or challenging time. Being listened to is about being recognized and being validated as a human being. It allows for the connection between people and reduces the feelings of loneliness and isolation. Sometimes it is easier to talk to a sympathetic and empathic stranger, such as a clinical or counselling psychologist, a psychotherapist or a counsellor, rather than to relatives or friends.

Some therapists will aim to help you find the root cause of your problems so that you can work out ways in which you might deal with the problems that have arisen as a result. This type of therapy is based on a psychodynamic or psychoanalytic approach. Some therapists may simply aim to listen to you and support you through creating a safe and consistent relationship and therapeutic environment in which to explore some of the difficulties you are facing. These may be trained in Rogerian Counselling or other forms of supportive therapy. There are also psychotherapists who use a combination of different therapeutic approaches; these are called integrative psychotherapists. Other therapists will help you to identify unhelpful behaviour or negative thinking patterns and together with you will then explore strategies to enable you to try out different, more helpful behaviour and more positive thinking patterns. These therapists would usually be trained in Cognitive Behavioural Psychotherapy (CBT). They would use therapeutic methods, which are similar to the approach this book is based on.

Sometimes, when some of your problems are related to specific traumas, possibly even traumas that happened early in life, then it could be helpful to work with therapists, who are trained in helping you to process and overcome the effects of these traumas. This would involve more than just talking about it. These therapists may be trained, sometimes additionally to their training in CBT or other forms of psychotherapy, in Eye Movement Desensitization and Reprocessing (EMDR). Both EMDR and CBT were approaches, which in 2005, were endorsed by the National Institute of Clinical Excellence (NICE) for being particularly effective therapies for the treatment of Posttraumatic Stress Disorder (PTSD), which often develops after trauma.

Clinical or Counselling Psychologists, Psychotherapists and Counsellors are trained to listen attentively and to support you to help you find your own answers, without judging you. The service they offer is confidential and they won't without your permission share any of the information you tell them with your partner or your friends.

You can get a referral made to a Clinical or Counselling Psychologist, a Psychotherapist or a Counsellor, usually through any of the health care professionals attached to your HIV service, most commonly your doctor. Most hospitals in the NHS already have Clinical or Counselling Psychologists, Counsellors or Psychotherapists attached to them who you can easily be referred to. Frequently, however, there is a waiting list and then you may have to wait a few weeks or sometimes even several months before you can be seen. In that case you may consider seeing a clinical psychologist, psychotherapist or counsellor privately.

If you want to contact a private Clinical or Counselling Psychologist, a Psychotherapist or a Counsellor you can contact the organisations listed in the Appendix. Usually, you will have to pay for their services. However, if you have a private health insurance it will be worth checking if they recognize your Clinical or Counselling Psychologist or Psychotherapist. In that case it may be that all or a part of your therapy will be paid for by your insurance. If you are thinking about seeking help privately, it will be important for you to check out the qualifications of any potential Psychologist, Psychotherapist or Counsellor. They should be registered with a professional organization and have a licensing certificate. If you are in doubt about anybody's appropriate qualifications you can make enquiries as to whether they are registered with their professional organization. Clinical and Counselling Psychologists, for example, have to be chartered and registered with the Health Professionals

Council (HPC). Psychotherapists also need to be accredited. One of these accrediting bodies, for example, is The United Kingdom Council for Psychotherapy (UKCP). Counsellors should also belong to a recognized accrediting body and you should check how long and with whom they have trained. It is important that they attended an accredited course, which should have spanned over a considerable amount of time not only a few weekends. In the Appendix section, we provide you with contact details for these organizations, who all have their own website of accredited members, from which you can choose a suitable Psychologist, Psychotherapist or Counsellor for you.

In order for you to benefit from any psychotherapy or counselling, whether you obtain this through the NHS or privately, it is important that you feel comfortable and safe with the professional you are seeing and that you find it easy to relate to them. It is important that they help you to develop a safe and trusting relationship with them. They need to be good at explaining things to you in a way that makes sense. It is also important that you feel comfortable about asking them questions that are important to you, such as, whether they have any experience of working with HIV issues, their attitude towards sexuality, race or gender or other areas of importance in your life. It is perfectly all right, also, for you to ask them about their qualifications and to explain to you their particular therapeutic approach.

If for any reason, you don't feel safe or comfortable with the professional you are seeing, you must raise this with them. If you feel that you can't raise it with them, it may be important for you to explore finding a different Clinical or Counselling Psychologist, Psychotherapist or Counsellor. Sometimes it is helpful, especially if you are seeking private treatment, to 'shop around' a bit. You may like to have an initial assessment consultation with a few professionals and then decide to work with the person who you felt most understood by and safe and comfortable with. It is important that you get this right.

# VOLUNTARY ORGANISATIONS AND SOCIAL SERVICES

Additionally to the health services you are entitled to, there are many other services available to you, such as benefit and housing advice. What is available may vary slightly from area to area or may be called differently. Ideally, each area should have access to the same range of services to address different levels of people's problems (such as, housing, benefits). If you call your local Council or Social Services and tell them what sort of services you are looking for then they will be able to direct you. You could also ask at your HIV clinic, as they should have good links with Social Services and other agencies in your area, especially as these may change throughout the course of your illness.

PART
A

PART
B

PART
C

SELF-MONITORING: A CHANCE TO CHECK-IN WITH YOURSELF • *Mental healthcare professionals (1) Have there been times when you have needed to talk to a professional (Counsellor, Psychologist, Psychotherapist, etc) about personal issues, fears or concerns? Do you experience any of these at the moment? Has a HIV diagnosis or ill health negatively affected you? Do you need to get back on track? (2) You might like to check-in with yourself to reflect on whether you know how you can access a professional if you needed them? It could be very helpful to write these down in your diary, notebook or on a sheet of paper, so that you can later decide on what might help you to tackle some of these.*

# CONCLUSION

There are many factors that can make it easier for you to negotiate an appropriate care network. These, in turn, will enhance your ability to be involved in your own care plan and to feel appropriately understood and supported. This will help you to cope better with your adherence to the various treatments that may be advised in your case. Therefore increasing the possibility that you can actively improve your quality of life. In order to be able to achieve this you will need to maintain regular contact with the hospital that monitors your HIV progress.

It is important that you feel some control over your care and know your network so that you can obtain help and be referred to the appropriate organisations when needed. It is important that you allow yourself to look after the care of your body and being HIV positive gives this need an even greater emphasis. You may consider seeking additional support with this, for example, through therapeutic massage or specific exercise classes, such as, Tai Chi or Yoga.

A balance of professional, voluntary and personal sources of support in negotiating your needs when living with HIV will help you immensely. We hope that the above assists you with examining and gaining greater understanding of how this balance is distributed in your current life with HIV and, also, enables you to identify any potential areas that could benefit from change in order to obtain an even better balance.

# HIV Disclosure and Challenging Stigma

# INTRODUCTION

Frequently an HIV positive diagnosis is unexpected and most people are unprepared. Even if the possibility has already been on a person's mind, having the diagnosis confirmed usually feels very different and brings up many new issues. As a result there is much that needs to be negotiated and thought about following an HIV positive diagnosis. This includes understanding how to live with HIV, reducing stress and negotiating care. Unfortunately, you may also experience shame and stigma in relation to having HIV, or you may hold fears about people judging you. This is because HIV has been associated with sex, disfigurement, death and many other socially taboo areas since its identification. These feelings may create a conflict in you as to whether and when to disclose in order to reach out for social support and also to whom and how to tell about your HIV positive diagnosis.

It can be a challenge to manage the task of disclosure to people outside your care network, such as, loved ones, family and friends. In the first instance it often requires for you to accept your HIV diagnosis in a non-judgemental way. This can be difficult, but is very important because it will help you to worry less about what others might think or how they will react. Also, whatever others think or how they might react, it will help you if you remain true to yourself and what you know to be right.

This chapter offers you an overview of some key issues in relation to helping you accept your diagnosis and some directions to help you think about disclosure.

# FACTORS THAT
# RELATE TO HIV/AIDS STIGMA

There are many factors that reinforce the stigma associated with HIV, which include that:

- HIV is a life threatening disease
- People are afraid of catching it
- The disease has been socially associated with already stigmatised behaviours such as injecting drugs and gay sex, and groups, such as homosexuals
- People living with HIV are often considered responsible for contracting the disease
- Moral or religious beliefs exist that regard HIV/AIDS as a deserving punishment for certain actions

PART
A

PART
B

PART
C

# MOTIVES FOR KEEPING SECRETS!

It is very common for many HIV+ people to keep secret about their HIV status. You cannot tell if someone is HIV+ just by looking at them so its presence remains hidden. The following five reasons may account for why you may not want to disclose your HIV status to others:

1 *TACT* to save the person you are telling embarrassment or upset
2 *RELATIONAL STABILITY* You may wish to avoid rejection or a difficult time with another person
3 *PSYCHOLOGICAL COMPENSATION* You may fear to lose your existing social status or image

4 *POWER DIFFERENTIAL* In order not to feel dependent
on acceptance from another person or inferior

5 *DENIAL* You may not be accepting of your diagnosis or recognize
the advantages of disclosure because of fear or depression

You may decide not to share your diagnosis at this stage, because you feel that it would be safer for you not to do so. If it is your decision not to disclose, it will be helpful for you to consider this carefully and have in your mind clear reasons as to why not. Equally, if you feel tempted to disclose, it is also important for you to be clear within yourself about the reasons for wanting to do so. It is a big step and once you have taken that step with a particular person, it will be a considerable investment and you will not be able to go back on it. Disclosure is important though and can have positive benefits, especially in relation to the people close to you.

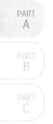

PART
A

PART
B

PART
C

# FACTORS RELATING TO HIV/AIDS ACCEPTANCE AND DISCLOSURE

We have covered some of the factors already, which will help you with adjusting better to your diagnosis. These related to your particular coping style, your problem solving skills, the way you think about the illness and its consequences, and your reactions to stress. We also considered in the last chapter the advantages of having positive, supportive social and professional relationships in order to help you adjust better. These will all assist you in the way in which you think about disclosure.

There are several advantages to disclosing your HIV status to another person, and research has demonstrated that, on the whole, people benefit from disclosure of emotional experiences to others. As can be seen in Figure (12), disclosure can be helpful. People have frequently given us the following reasons for their disclosure: the wish

---

**WHY HIV DISCLOSURE IS IMPORTANT**

- DISCLOSURE is easier in the long run as it is hard to keep important personal information secret from people close to you.
- DISCLOSURE can help with your adaptation to illness by enabling others to support you with the processing of disturbing emotions, and problem solving.
- DISCLOSURE to care staff can lead to access to specialist treatment.
- DISCLOSURE can help you access practical and emotional help in the longer term.
- DISCLOSURE can help you overcome loneliness.
- DISCLOSURE can help you overcome feeling that you are the only one with the condition and your potential fears of stigma.
- DISCLOSURE can help to change attitudes in those around you.
- DISCLOSURE can wake others up to the fact that HIV is a global phenomenon, as it can affect anyone, whoever they are and where ever they live in this world.

PART
A

PART
B

PART
C

**Fig. 12**  Why HIV disclosure is important

---

to avoid negative consequences, such as: illness; people finding out and feeling betrayed, rather than being told; preventing the spread of HIV; in order to improve the situation for themselves or others, such as being able to obtain more support and recognition of their difficulties; and in order not to be so lonely with the knowledge of having the condition of HIV.

*Mavis' was afraid to tell her partner after she found out in the antenatal clinic that she was positive, because she feared her partner would reject her. After the delivery she needed more help than ever to be able to deal with her life and was finding it hard to keep such a big secret, while she was also dealing with her emotions related to the birth of her new baby and her positive status. She decided to tell her partner. He was shocked at first and then sad, but when he realized that there were treatments available so that Mavis could still have a future and they could spend their future life together, and that it would not affect the health of their baby, and he tested negative, their relationship continued and Mavis received the support she needed.*

PART
A

PART
B

PART
C

However, despite the possible advantages of disclosing your HIV status to others, as in Mavis' case, it often takes much thought, planning and perseverance due to possible fears of the response you might get from others, as a result of stigma or prejudices. You may be concerned about social rejection, exclusion, abandonment, anger, violence and emotional withdrawal, and many other people in your position have felt that way.

Unfortunately, in a few cases these fears are justified. It is therefore important that you allow yourself time to consider who to disclose to and when to disclose. You may want to reflect carefully on what you know about the person you may want to disclose to. What is their general attitude toward HIV and how have you known them to be talking about other people's difficulties or problems in the past? It may also be important to plan how you will disclose and deal with the possible reactions of others. You may want to be aware of what other stressors are going on for them in their life and evaluate carefully when it would feel right to disclose.

Due to the conflict you may be feeling about these considerations, you may delay your actual disclosure. However in our experience, circumstances, such as illness and taking combination therapy, have made people disclose in the end. Often it helps enormously to be released from the load of carrying your problems on your own, despite the initial experience of other people's reactions to your condition.

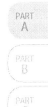

# WHAT MAY HELP
# IF YOU ARE DECIDING TO DISCLOSE?

There are many possible situations and people you could have to make the decision to disclose your HIV status to. This could include situations where it may appear that you have less choice, such as:

- Health and social care professionals in order to receive medical or social care and support
- Employers where it is required for you to disclose a "disability" on the application form
- Insurance companies when applying for mortgages or travel insurance
- Immigration when considering travelling to certain countries that require HIV disclosure

However, in this section we will consider those important decisions you will need to make with:

- Your partner, close friends, family, or your community

*SELF-MONITORING: A CHANCE TO CHECK-IN WITH YOURSELF • HIV disclosure (1) How comfortable do you feel about being HIV+? How accepting are you of your diagnosis? Have any of these thoughts and feelings changed since you were diagnosed for the better or worse? What can account for these changes? Do you ever feel you will fully accept being HIV+? (2) Using this chapter, think about your 'disclosure'. Who have you disclosed to, why and how did you do it? Do you think that you should tell more people or are you happy with whom you have told so far? It could be very helpful to make some notes about the above in your diary, notebook or on a sheet of paper, so that you can later decide on what might help you to take some of your observations further.*

# (1) BEING MORE ACCEPTING OF HAVING HIV

To start with we have suggested that it is important to establish how much you yourself accept having HIV. Identifying and challenging your own beliefs about the HIV stigma is an important step toward psychological acceptance of having HIV. For example, if you believe that you are to blame for getting HIV then it will be harder for you to accept it or tell others. In this context, it is very important to distinguish between regret and blame. It is perfectly natural to regret getting HIV, and perhaps you will always feel some regret. But blaming yourself is very different, as it often involves harsh self-criticism and feeling a failure, and you can end up believing that because you became HIV positive, you no longer deserve good things in your life.

Depending on your particular circumstances, you may feel that you are not responsible for contracting HIV. However, it may equally be that, reflecting on your situation, you decide that you are partially and sometimes even fully responsible for contracting HIV. Even if you decide that you are fully responsible for contracting HIV, it is important that you do not blame yourself. Blame is a very damaging and unhelpful emotion, which keeps you trapped in a negative loop of self-punishment. If you experience a lot of feelings of self-blame, which you find you can't shift, it could be very helpful to consult a HIV Counsellor, a Clinical Psychologist or a Psychotherapist about this.

Another feeling that you may encounter could be shame. Internal shame relates to your own feelings and beliefs about your perceived 'difference' in comparison to others or the attitudes you carry inside yourself about that 'difference'. These can range from self-acceptance to self-hatred. Can you try to identify some of your own feelings in relation to this? It may be helpful to write them down and acknowledge them in that way. Figure (13) shows an Acceptance Continuum. Where do you feel you are on this at this present moment in time?

PART
A

PART
B

PART
C

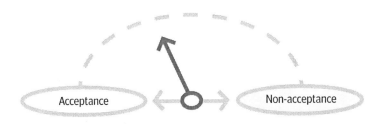

**Fig. 13** HIV acceptance continuum

Figure (14) lists questions for you to ask yourself in relation to your own feelings of self-acceptance of having HIV. By working through the questions you may find out about areas that would be useful for you to address in order to help you build your self-acceptance.

What are your thoughts and feelings about having HIV? Are they accepting or regretful? Are they upsetting or negative or positive?

Explore possible reasons behind these feelings and thoughts (for example: personal, such as the circumstances of how you contracted HIV; your cultural values, such as associations with African people; stigma; or fear of other people's reactions, etc).

Write down the positive and negative impact of your feelings and thoughts about having HIV on your life (for example: it made you make positive changes in your life as a result, which you would otherwise not have done; or it brought up unpleasant feelings of isolation in you, etc).

Try and look at evidence for any negative beliefs you may have about having HIV, for example, that no one will like you again, and think about whether someone who you trust and who's opinion you value, would share your beliefs.

Check whether your beliefs about having HIV have changed the way you see yourself and whether your self worth is for the better or worse.

If you have not already done so, think about how disclosing HIV has affected your social interactions. What have the negative and what have the positive aspects been for you, as a result of your self-disclosure?

PART
A

PART
B

PART
C

**Fig. 14** How self accepting are you?

# (2) BEING MORE SELF-ACCEPTING

The more accepting about having HIV, and the more confident you are, the easier it will be to help another important person in your life to come to terms with your condition. Remember, having HIV is a condition that has now become part of your life, however, it is not the whole of your identity and it does not make you a less worthy person. Comparing yourself to others who are not affected by HIV or who seem to be better off in relation to their HIV, is usually not helpful. You are only hurting yourself with such thoughts, and this will further increase your suffering, rather than reducing it as much as possible. The following exercise may help you to start thinking about other valuable aspects of yourself that you may have lost sight of, as a result of your HIV diagnosis.

It is common, especially at the early stages of the diagnosis, to be completely preoccupied by your HIV. It may feel as if everything else in life has lost its significance for you. However, the diagram in Figure (15) wants to remind you that there are many aspects that shape your

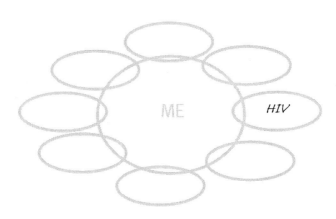

**Fig. 15** My identity

identity and that having HIV is one aspect. Please add to the diagram other things that shape your identity that you feel are important, such as, the particular qualities you hold as a person, activities and skills you are good at, relationships you have, any work you do, where you come from, your social roles, such as daughter, son or wife, and so forth. Allow yourself to recognize the importance of all those aspects, too.

## (3) ANSWERING "SHOULD I?" OR "SHOULD I NOT?" QUESTIONS

PART
A

PART
B

PART
C

You may then like to do the following exercise in Figure (16). Please write in the 'for' column all the reasons why right now or at a certain time in the future you might like to disclose your status to a particular person in your life, and in the 'against' column the reasons why not. Then work out if the 'for' outweigh the 'against' arguments. You can now start to work out some of the conditions you may be able to change, in order for you to be ready to disclose your HIV status. If you are not ready to disclose to this person at this moment in time, you could always come back and do this exercise at a later time to find out what your position is then. You can also use this exercise for evaluating who the people are with whom you feel safe to disclose to at this stage, and with whom you do not.

## (4) MAKING A PLAN

After your evaluation of the various factors that speak for or against disclosure, you may then decide to disclose or decide to wait until

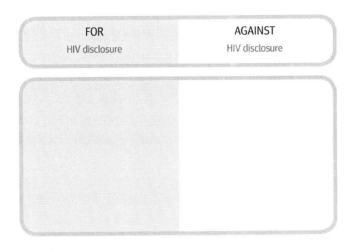

| FOR HIV disclosure | AGAINST HIV disclosure |
| --- | --- |
|  |  |

Fig. 16   Working out the pros and cons of HIV disclosure

PART
A

PART
B

PART
C

certain conditions are fulfilled. For example, you may decide to tell a parent only when you are ill, or a friend only if you are going on holiday with them while you are on combination therapies.

If you do decide to disclose, it will be helpful for you to plan when, how, and the type of follow up you will have, before you take any action. It is best to have thought about this carefully, rather than acting out of impulse by disclosing in a certain situation, which you may later regret. Before you disclose, it could be helpful for you to think through a few more issues. One is that it is not possible to predict exactly or control how people will react. It is helpful therefore for you to expect that most people, whom you tell, will initially experience some sense of shock, especially, as they are likely to have some caring or loving feelings about you. They may go through similar feelings to the ones you went through when you first found out and worry that your life will be shorter. Therefore, however the person you disclose to responds, please remember that it may take some time for them to really come to terms with what you have told them and you may need to follow their path to acceptance. Be prepared to support them through this path, before expecting that you may feel supported by them. Whilst we can't say that everyone you tell will accept your diagnosis, it is important to remember that no one has the right to abuse or hurt you physically or mentally, and that if they do you must avoid them or get help, if this is not possible.

The second issue that could be helpful for you to think through is to imagine for yourself what the very worst response could be that you could be getting from a particular person in response to your HIV disclosure. Imagine the worst things that they could be saying to you and then imagine if that really happened, how you would respond. Imagine how you would cope if that really happened. Imagine further, if they really did respond in that way, what would that say about them and your relationship to them? Also, think if they really responded in that very worst way, whether, knowing them, you think that this would only be their initial response, as a result of their shock, or do you feel that their attitude wouldn't change with time? If they really responded in that very worst way, how would you feel about them as your friends or as someone you would want close to you during times of need? Imagine, if they really responded in that way and stayed with those very worst responses, how you would cope? Imagine what action you would take to get over it and come to terms with their reaction? Make a plan for yourself of how you would protect yourself and what other resources or people you would draw on if that really happened. If you can do all that, you are ready to disclose.

Your disclosure may not be easy. It is a *process* and not a one-off event. Prepare yourself that if the person you wish to tell has not been

PART
A

PART
B

PART
C

expecting or contemplating the possibility of you having contracted HIV, the disclosure may come as an enormous shock to them. It takes thought, planning and self-acceptance. Additionally, you need to prepare yourself to help someone else to go through the stages of coming to terms with your diagnosis in similar ways to the ones that you experienced. Because of the work involved, it could be wise not to disclose to too many people at the same time. Initially, you need to be giving much more to the other person than they can give to you. You have the advantage of having known your condition for some time. You can get support and coaching for preparing for your disclosure from your health care team. For example, they may set up a meeting to help you tell someone of importance to you if you feel that kind of support could be of help to you. Also, it may be helpful for you to let them know of your intention so that they can support you during your process of disclosure.

Chapter (10) provides you with an example of problem-solved disclosure to help you think about how to negotiate whom to tell.

PART
A

PART
B

PART
C

# (5) AVOIDING AND OVERCOMING LONELINESS

If you do decide to do it alone and end up not disclosing, one of the consequences may be loneliness. This can result in feeling cut off and depressed. The following tips may help you in dealing with this:

## (1) Recognize your own Thinking Patterns.

When your mood is low there is a tendency for your thinking to become quite negative. Often this is because the way in which you perceive things during these times is not the way in which things actually are in reality. We call this pattern of thinking – distorted thinking. It includes 'all-or-nothing' thinking or exaggerated thinking, during which you blow things out of their actual proportion or context. You can recognize this pattern of thinking because of its catastrophic and absolute nature. Here are some examples of common thoughts associated with loneliness: *"I have no friends!; "No one likes or loves me!"; "What good am I to anybody?; "Nobody understands me"; "I am completely undesirable"; "I have no value whatsoever in society!"*.

Upon reading these, explore what your thinking patterns are and if some of your thoughts might also be distorted. Chapter 9 looks at HIV-related cognitive distortions in more detail and ways to change your thoughts. You may at this stage try and identify some thoughts that you have found yourself thinking in relation to your own possible feelings of loneliness. It could be helpful for you to write these down.

## (2) Stop Comparing Yourself with Others

A common problem is that we often compare ourselves with others who have what we think we want, need or desire. The pattern is that we focus on a particular aspect in another person's life, where we think that other person has an advantage over us. However, there are big problems with comparing ourselves.

Firstly, it can never be accurate. This is because usually we will only ever focus on a small part of that other person's life in our comparison. We leave out all the other areas, which this person may, in actual fact, struggle with. We make the assumption that because the particular area of our focus seems okay for that other person (and this is still only based on our perception, because it may not actually feel okay for the other person), the rest of their life must also be okay. Of course, when we do that, we don't take into account that person's whole reality. There may be many things that we don't know about or which we can't see about this person that makes them feel quite different to how we perceive it. Therefore our perception that things are better for another person are purely based on our assumptions, but may not at all reflect the reality for that other person.

Secondly, we are all unique. Every one of us comes with their own particular talents, their personality and their own, unique life experiences and each person has their own strengths and weaknesses and purpose in life. Comparison only works if two things are exactly the same and then we can decide which one of the two is actually better. When you compare yourself with another person, you are never comparing two equals and therefore this comparison can never be accurate and is in actual fact very unfair to yourself. It makes you discount your own path and what life challenges you had to master to get to where you are at this stage in your life.

Thirdly, when we make comparisons, we usually think in a very judgemental way about ourselves, whereby we assume that what the other people do is usually better and what we do is bad, undesirable or worthless. Therefore we are judging ourselves negatively on something that we aren't actually really in a position to judge. We are hurting ourselves and putting ourselves down with something that is solely based on our assumption rather than actual reality. This then makes us feel bad and reinforces our feelings of loneliness and isolation.

Here are some common examples of comparison with others: *"Everyone is busier and happier than me"; "Everybody else has fulfilling relationships"; "Others with HIV infection have much better friendship networks"; "Everybody is clearer about the focus and purpose in their life than me!"; "The doctor who advised me on my medication today,*

PART
A

PART
B

PART
C

*has so much of a better life than me; He so much more social and at
ease than me!"* Allow yourself to explore whether you also compare
yourself with others. Identify some of the assumptions you might be
making about other people's lives and their relationships in comparison
to your own. You may like to write this down. As we explored above,
by thinking in this way, you put yourself into an impossible situation,
which does not do justice to where you actually are in your own life at
this point, because it is not only unfair but also based on incorrect and
biased assumptions.

## (3) Recognize the Vicious Spiral of Low Mood

Notice how your own mood can lead to you withdrawing from other
people because of your fear of being hurt or rejected by them. It is
a common problem that when we feel low we withdraw from other
people, even our friends, and we may even push them away. This is
not at all helpful because it is during these times when we especially
need contact and need the comfort of that closeness. You might like
to try and turn this process around. Make yourself aware of how you
currently feel and ask yourself what your true needs are. Are your
needs really for loneliness and withdrawal? Or are they really for
comfort, warmth and closeness? Don't be frightened of admitting your
needs to yourself.

Once you have admitted these feelings to yourself and may be
even written them down in your journal, try and verbalize them to your
friends. You could start approaching others rather than avoiding them.
You could plan activities that increase your social contacts. You could
contact people you know and like. You could talk to neighbours. You
could develop a hobby, which might provide you with some positive
occupation and help you establish new contacts.

PART
A

PART
B

PART
C

## (4) Recognize the Difference
## between Being Alone and Loneliness

It is a common error that we equate being alone with loneliness. Most of us don't like the feelings of loneliness, which may be based also on how we experienced loneliness when we were young and when we most needed continuous and permanent access to contact. As a result, in order to avoid these unpleasant feelings, we may also avoid being alone. However, being alone doesn't mean that we have to be lonely. It is important that we all learn to enjoy being in our own company. Learn to enjoy doing things and caring for yourself on your own. Cook yourself a nice meal, play your favourite music, read a good book. The more you can feel at home with yourself – not looking around for others all the time – the more confident and internally strong a person you will become. When you are doing things for yourself on your own, be mindful of using a positive and encouraging language and attitude towards yourself about what you are doing. It is important for you to learn to be kind and accepting of yourself.

Allow yourself to identify your own feelings about being on your own. Is it something that comes easy to you and is pleasurable or do you avoid it because it is unpleasant? Try and explore your own relationship to yourself. Identify what you might do to develop a more caring and nurturing attitude toward yourself, so that it will be comfortable for you to stay in your own company.

PART A

PART B

PART C

## (5) Plan a Variety of
## Satisfying Activities to do on your Own

Enjoying your own company can include planning satisfying activities you enjoy and feel in control of, which in turn can improve your mood. Examples include going to an art gallery or walking in the park. Use your imagination. Before you carry out an activity draw up a chart and rate how satisfying you think a particular activity will be for you to do on a scale of 0-100 (0= no satisfaction, 100= enormous satisfaction). Then after you have carried out the activity, rate the actual satisfaction that you have felt. Identify the factors that have provided you with satisfaction and consider whether you could do activities that include those factors. Notice also what was difficult for you to do and explore what might help you to overcome these difficulties. Plan what you might want to try doing differently when you do your next activity. Listen to your own needs and what feels good to you.

## (6) List Some Advantages of Being Alone.

It is important for you to learn to appreciate the value of 'time alone'. This is special time with yourself and allows you *an opportunity to explore how you really feel and think.* This may initially be a bit scary for you. In fact, you may have avoided being on your own, because you don't want to face how you really feel and think. While your fear is understandable, it is important that you realize that if you don't know how you feel or think, you cannot be in control of yourself. In order to make decisions that are good for you, feel right for you and meet your needs, you need to know how you feel and think. If you feel this is a real obstacle for you, it maybe that counselling or psychotherapy might help you to find ways of learning to recognize how you feel and think.

Another advantage of being alone sometimes is that it allows you to develop greater personal strength. You may like to become aware of why you may have avoided spending time alone before. Often people avoid spending time being on their own, because that way they don't have to face up to what they really feel, which may be painful. Essentially, this prevents a person from knowing who they really are and what is important for them in their life. Being on your own and learning to feel comfortable with this can be like coming home to yourself.

**SELF-MONITORING: A CHANCE CHECK-IN WITH YOURSELF** • *Loneliness ( I ) Have you ever felt lonely because of being HIV +? Have you ever felt more isolated because of being HIV+? (2) How have you managed your feelings of isolation? Think about the difference between being alone and loneliness. Have you ever used any of the tips suggested here for overcoming loneliness? It could be very helpful to make some notes about the above in your diary, notebook or on a sheet of paper, so that you can later decide on what might help you to take some of your observations further.*

PART
A

PART
B

PART
C

# CONCLUSION

There are many personal factors that relate to HIV stigma, to HIV disclosure and acceptance, such as your beliefs and experiences. As we have acknowledged, having HIV is a health problem that can produce difficult emotions and situations when you disclose to another person. Nevertheless, sometimes it is the best thing to disclose and at other times it is not. The choice ultimately has to be yours but it is helpful for you to have spent some time consciously thinking through the reasons behind your decision. In addition to the suggestions we make in this book, you can also receive professional help to support you with working out whether to disclose and how to do it.

It is important, if you are not able to tell people about your status at present, that you watch out for not becoming too isolated as this can make you feel worse and even less inclined to disclose in the longer term. Disclosure is an important issue for most people with HIV. Remember that there are increasing numbers of people still being infected by HIV today. You are not on your own in that there will be many people in your position. You might like to remind yourself, when you are considering your choices about disclosure, that successful coping with HIV involves living well in the present and you might like to let that guide you in your decision.

# 5

# Sexual Relationships
# and HIV

# INTRODUCTION

This chapter provides information to help HIV positive people in their sexual lives. It is written for both sexes, different cultures, gay, bisexual and heterosexuals alike and should be useful regardless of the type of sexual relationships you engage in. It will outline ways HIV can affect sexual functioning and relationships and discuss issues relating to safer sex and HIV positive people. It will also explore some ways in which people think about sex and outline facts about sex and causes of sexual problems. Additionally, an overview of the importance of communication in sexual relationships will be provided.

PART
A

PART
B

PART
C

# IMPACT OF HIV ON SEX AND RELATIONSHIPS

The association between HIV and sex has unfortunately often been portrayed negatively. Since sexually transmitted infections were identified thousands of years ago, different groups of people have always been stigmatised. For example, at the end of the last century the English regarded syphilis as a French disease and the French regarded it as an English disease! The stigma around HIV made it harder for people to feel they were entitled to a satisfying sexual and relationship life. Some reductions in stigma and discrimination, together with an increased life expectancy mean that this is changing. More and more HIV positive people are thinking about and engaging in sex and relationships and are determined to reintroduce positive experiences into their life.

HIV can affect sexual functioning in many ways. It is quite common for people when first diagnosed to lose their sexual interest and desire. This can be related to many things but common reasons include:

- Fear of passing the virus on to others
- Distress associated with the diagnosis
- Guilt and shame about how it was contracted
  and what others will think
- Concerns about catching other sexually transmitted
  infections (STI's)

This may also have applied or may still apply to you. However, you may find that over time as you adjust to your diagnosis, your sexual interest and desire returns. You maybe able to experience satisfying sexual relationships, but you may also have some sexual difficulties, such as problems with erections or orgasm. The factors associated with sexual problems in HIV positive people are discussed later in this chapter, but they can impact upon your relationships, such as, by making you avoid meeting new partners or affecting the level of intimacy you experience within your relationships.

HIV can also influence the non-sexual side of your relationship. You might avoid meeting people for fear of rejection. It can also affect the way you relate to a partner. Specifically, it may affect the roles each of you takes in relation to the other. For example, the person diagnosed with HIV will need more "caring" than the other (regardless of their own status), temporarily. Equally, your partner may protect you from their feelings out of fear of overburdening you during a difficult time. HIV may also affect how you see yourself. It will therefore also influence the way in which you believe other people will see you. This is likely to include the way in which you feel about your own attractiveness and lovability. You may feel so undesirable that you are pushing people away, who are potentially loving and understanding toward you. HIV can have a devastating effect on your self-image in this way.

PART
A

PART
B

PART
C

# HIV AND SAFER SEX

The rate of new HIV infections continues to increase. This reflects, at least in part, the number of people practising unsafe sex. Researchers have suggested many reasons for this. For example, it is not surprising that people do not use condoms 100% of the time. This can be due to many factors, such as pressures from a partner not to use a condom; skill factors around putting condoms on; reduced consciousness as a result of different mental states (such as intoxication or drugs); misperceptions about safety without condoms; reduced penile sensation; lack of control during situations of sexual excitement; and so on. People rarely achieve a 100% level of perfection in terms of their use of condoms. It is increasingly recognised, however, that not using a condom or using a condom inconsistently puts people at significant risk, which is reflected by the increase in rates of new HIV infections.

Some people, such as gay men who are HIV positive, use a strategy, referred to as "negotiated safety". This involves disclosing your own HIV status and only having sex without condoms when your sexual partner is also known to be HIV positive and agrees to have unprotected sex. Medically this is not risk free, as there is the chance of contracting new drug resistant strains of HIV or other STI's. However, there is evidence that negotiated safety has become of some value within some sections of the HIV positive community.

Some sociologists have viewed negotiated safety as a way in which HIV positive gay men are taking control of their sex lives. If you are engaging in this practice or are considering doing it, it is worth thinking about the potential risks involved and asking yourself if you are prepared to live with the negative costs, which 'negotiated safety' might entail. Ultimately, you are responsible for making choices and for carrying consequences, which you feel you can live with. You might consider carefully what kind of sexual activity is safe enough for you and compare this with the safety information available.

You may find yourself in a situation in which you would like to use condoms, because they are safer, but find it difficult to use them at all or consistently. This is not an uncommon problem and it can be quite distressing. Possible reasons for non-use might include that some men find they lose their erection when trying to use condoms. Therefore they avoid using them in order to reduce the likelihood of erectile failure. Also, it takes some practice to put condoms on skilfully so that they work and sit comfortably. This may need to be learned and practiced in the same way as you would with any other new skill.

Another reason why condoms are not used may relate to power differences in some relationships. For example, in some communities men have historically played a dominant role over women and this can make it difficult for women to exert their need for a man to use condoms in sexual relationships. While it would be very important for the woman to be protected, the man may not have learned to consider and take her needs into account, and may expose her to risk of infection. Some men can find it very frustrating when they are limited in exercising their sexual desires freely, because of the need to protect themselves or their sexual partner.

If you find that you are in this category and you feel frustrated and possibly even sometimes assert your will onto another person, it is important that you start to really think about the consequences of your actions. This is because engaging in unprotected sex compromises your own and the other person's safety and health. Is this really what you want? Are you really prepared to carry the consequences and be accountable for your actions? If you are already HIV positive, do you

PART
A

PART
B

PART
C

feel that it is fair or ethical to expose another person to the same risk? Allow yourself to question your motivation for engaging in such an action. You may not usually think about these consequences during times when you engage in sexual behaviour that puts others at risk. You may block out the longer-term consequences in moments of potential sexual pleasure.

In the United Kingdom, there have been several prosecutions in recent years of HIV positive people for, what the legal system refers to as "the reckless" transmission of HIV to their sexual partners, also known as biological grievous bodily harm (GBH). In other countries, such as Canada and Australia, there have also been small increases in the number of these prosecutions. In almost all cases it has involved positive people in long-term relationships where the Court has heard evidence that the HIV positive person declined to use condoms and offered false reassurances to their partner that they were HIV negative. We are against any moves to criminalise HIV transmission, because we believe this would make it even harder for HIV positive people to disclose their status because of fear of prosecution, and fails to recognise the discrimination and stigma experienced by HIV positive people in their everyday lives. It is understandable that hearing about such cases could have left you feeling worried. However, we feel that it is important to raise this issue to inform you, rather than alarm you, because we feel these prosecutions are something you need to be aware of. You can access advice and information about this issue from the Terence Higgins Trust, and the websites listed at the end of this book. In any case your best protection is to always wear a condom and inform all your sexual partners of your status.

Maybe this book will help you to start expanding your framework of thinking around these issues that does not only consider the short-lived pleasures of the moment, but moves toward understanding and considering the potential long-term consequences of your actions, which unprotected sexual behaviour may have on another person.

There are many other potential reasons for why men are not using a condom and it is not always clear to people which may apply to them. If you are finding it difficult to use condoms and this is putting others at risk, you can always discuss the issue in confidence with staff at your Sexual Health Centre or HIV clinic, such as Clinical Psychologists or Health Advisers. They can help you identify and address the factors, which are preventing you from engaging in safe sex, and explore the use of more helpful and safe sexual practises with you.

# MYTHS ABOUT SEX

There are many myths about sex. In this context it is worth asking yourself how you first learnt what you know about sex. For most people it is unlikely that this would have been through sex education at school. Instead it is more likely to have been through trial and error in the sexual relationships you have had and from sources, like erotic magazines or films. People spend a lot of time talking about sex in different forms, with each other, in newspapers and magazines, and on television. Much of this talk focuses on how well (or how badly) people perform during sexual encounters. You may have also asked yourself this question at some point in your life. The problem is that you may have had to rely on word of mouth or erotic films to compare yourself with others. To a large extent these unofficial sources contain a number of "myths". Bernard Zilbergeld, a Psychologist and Sexologist, identified several common sexual myths found in society.

PART
A

PART
B

PART
C

For example:

- sexual activity should always involve penetration
- sex always requires a constant erection
- good sex requires spontaneity
- women must always come to orgasm

If you have HIV, there are many new faulty beliefs in circulation that can get in the way of satisfying sexual relationships. Do you hold any unhelpful beliefs in your mind in relation to having HIV? Some of the new 'myths' in circulation are, listed, below. For example:

PART
A

PART
B

PART
C

- that HIV makes you less attractive
- that you cannot have children if you are HIV positive
- that you are dangerous and that you will
  easily transmit the virus during sex

It is not uncommon for people to disconnect the physical aspects of sex from the emotional and psychological aspects. You may be used to thinking of your sexual organs as somehow separate from the rest of your body. You may also think that they should be fully operational at all times, regardless of your psychological or emotional condition. You may be surprised to discover that arousal (e.g. erections in men, vaginal lubrication in women) usually stems from cognitive (thinking) activity in the brain, not just from local stimulation. The point is that you are not a machine when it comes to sex. What is happening in your mind at the time is also of crucial importance. Therefore, if you find yourself having negative beliefs about your sexual functioning in relation to being HIV positive it might be worth checking out the validity of these beliefs. You may discover that you are very unkind and unfair to yourself. You might find it helpful to read more about this in the section on problems with sexual functioning. If your negative thoughts about yourself or your self-image in relation to your HIV are so distressing that you can't shift them and they interfere in your ability to enjoy sex, you may benefit from talking to a Clinical Psychologist, who may be able to help you to feel more comfortable with and accepting of yourself.

## MYTHS ABOUT HIV INFECTION DURING SEX AND RELATIONSHIPS

There are in addition many misconceptions and myths about how HIV can be contracted. However, there are only four main routes by which HIV can be transmitted:

- Through unprotected vaginal or anal sex, whatever your sexuality
- By sharing needles, if you are injecting drugs, receiving a tattoo or any other procedure involving the shared use of needles
- Mother to baby during pregnancy, birth, or through breastfeeding
- Through infected blood or blood products, as part of a medical treatment. In the UK the chances of this happening is remote as all the blood, blood products and donated organs are screened for HIV and infected materials destroyed.

It cannot be transmitted by:

- Kissing
- Touching and holding hands

- Sharing eating utensils
- Toilet seats
- Insect or animal bites
- Swimming pools
- Breathing over someone
- Using the same towel as someone with HIV
- Talking to someone

During sex the best way to prevent transmission is to use a condom each and every time you have anal or vaginal sex. Oral sex where one partner uses their tongue or mouth to stimulate their partner's genitals poses a very low risk of HIV transmission and can be further reduced by:

- Avoiding getting semen or pre-ejaculatory fluid in the mouth, particularly if there are any cuts, sores or ulcers in the mouth
- Using a condom for oral sex with a man or a dental dam (a latex square) for oral sex with a woman.

SELF-MONITORING: A CHANCE TO CHECK-IN WITH YOURSELF • *being sexual and HIV+* (1) *How did you relate to sex before you were diagnosed HIV+? How did you express your sexuality before your diagnosis? (2) since you have been diagnosed HIV+ how has your sex life changed? What does 'sex' and being 'sexual' mean to you now? It could be helpful to make some notes about the above in your diary, notebook or on a sheet of paper, so that you can later decide on what might help you to take some of your observations further.*

PART
A

PART
B

PART
C

# THE HUMAN SEXUAL RESPONSE

In order to create a framework for understanding problems with sexual functioning it will be helpful to consider the normal sexual response, which is shared by all human beings.

The human sexual response shown in Figure (17) illustrates the psychological and physical responses to sex. Usually, during sexual encounters a person goes through four different phases:

The human sexual response can seem quite complex. The above demonstrates that it involves four phases and therefore an awareness of each of these phases and what each entails can make it easier for you to understand. Knowing of what to expect may make you feel more relaxed

PART
A

PART
B

PART
C

**(1) APPETITE**
This phase is when you start deciding that you are in the mood for sex. You may feel that you want sex or you know that you are going to engage in it. Before you become aroused you need an appetite. Both men and women are largely the same in terms of their needs at this phase. However, there are differences in terms of the types of appetites that people have.

**(2) AROUSAL or EXCITEMENT**
In men, erection of the penis may be the first thing to happen. As arousal is increased, he feels more excited, breathes more heavily and may feel tense and sweaty. In women, slight swelling of the outer lips of the vagina and increased lubrication inside the vagina occur at this early stage of arousal.

**Fig. 17** The human sexual response (cont. on next page)

**(3) CLIMAX or ORGASM**

Increase in arousal can be achieved through many ways and depends on personal preferences. Many women enjoy having their clitoris caressed. As arousal increases, the man reaches a point after which there is no return to a lesser state of arousal and he will ejaculate, whatever happens. The fluid ejaculated can vary in quality and quantity but it is usually about a teaspoonful. As he ejaculates he experiences a climax, which is a sudden build up and release of tension followed by a feeling of well-being and calm.

**(4) RESOLUTION**

This is like the lull after the storm. The body settles down and both partners feel fulfilled and calm, often pleasantly sleepy and relaxed. In the woman the feeling of fullness or congestion in her pelvis and her general sense of excitement may take longer to settle than in the man, particularly if she has not experienced a climax as part of the sexual encounter.

and therefore might allow you to explore what satisfies your needs in each of these phases and enable you to feel more sexual pleasure.

# WHY SEXUAL PROBLEMS ARISE

Sex is a natural function like digestion. Just like digestion it can be upset by a whole variety of problems, not just physical factors. We all expect that an unhealthy eating style, such as feeling rushed, stressed, anxious or in a bad mood while eating, can lead to complaints like loss of appetite, indigestion, diarrhoea or constipation even though our body is basically healthy. We also know that if we eat in a relaxed manner and can enjoy our food, our appetite and digestive system work well. In a similar way, if sex is allowed to happen naturally and in a relaxed atmosphere our bodies will respond normally without any conscious effort on our part.

You may find that you are experiencing sexual problems. Sexual problems are extremely common. Around forty percent of the adult population will experience sexual problems at some point in their lives. It is also known that people with HIV experience sexual problems more commonly than others. This is because sexual behaviour is determined by a host of biological and psychological influences that can be adversely affected by HIV. Therefore, many people with HIV are suffering from some form of sexual problem.

PART
A

PART
B

PART
C

People have been concerned about the possible part that Antiretrovirals may play in causing sexual problems amongst HIV positive people, particularly erectile problems in men. While Antiretrovirals (and HIV itself) can directly cause sexual problems the rate of sexual problems in people with HIV does not seem to have significantly risen since the introduction of antiretroviral medication. Additionally, it is difficult for research to exactly measure cause and effect, because with the advent of antiretroviral medication people with HIV were able to live longer and therefore some of the sexual problems could also be due to other factors, such as new psychological or environmental stressors arising from this. Therefore rather than relying on generalized research, it is more helpful to carefully assess for each person, which factors may cause their particular sexual problems. This can be done through careful assessment by appropriately trained professionals, such as your Medical Consultant, a Clinical Psychologist, a Health Advisor, and others, depending on their particular experience and training in this area.

If you do have any sexual problems, such as erectile problems or reduced sexual desire, it would be helpful to find out who in your particular HIV service may be able to do such an assessment with you. Sometimes, you may have to meet with several different professionals to explore the different factors that may be involved.

The possible factors (both general and HIV specific) that can be involved in sexual problems are listed below. You may like to assess if any of them affect you at the moment.

PART
A

PART
B

PART
C

# 1.BIOLOGICAL

## GENERAL HEALTH

Poor health influences sexual ability significantly. Appetite for sex, like appetite for food, often (though not always) goes away when you have been ill or had an accident. It rebuilds gradually as you regain your physical health. Therefore, it will be important for you that you allow your body to be as healthy as it can be. Good drug adherence will be a factor that helps to maintain your physical health. Other aspects will be a healthy diet and appropriate exercise.

However, some of the side effects of HIV medications can make it harder for a person to feel the desire for sex. For example, lipodystrophy (fatty redistributions in the body) can occur as a result of taking some combination drugs. This can make people feel less attractive and this may reduce their desire to engage in sex. If this does affect you it could be helpful to explore some of the negative perceptions you have about yourself with your doctor or another professional, who may be able to help you with this.

## NEUROLOGICAL

Unfortunately, sometimes HIV can damage neural structures in the region of the brain, spinal cord or peripheral nerve pathways, which relate to experiencing sexual sensations. This can reduce your ability to feel sexual sensation.

## VASCULAR

Adequate blood flow and pressure is needed for you to experience a sexual response in the genital area. This can be disrupted by any illness, for example arterial disease, which is often caused by smoking. Your body will have a lot to deal with carrying the HIV. Therefore, you might like to explore whether to adjust your lifestyle and give up any substances, like nicotine, which add further burden on your physical system.

## HORMONAL

The hormone most commonly associated with low sexual desire is testosterone. This can be low in some people with HIV as a result of physical changes and stress. However, cognitive factors can override the influence of hormonal aspects of sexual functioning. This means that it is possible, if you have positive thoughts in relation to yourself and your situation, to override some of the effects that the hormones might otherwise have.

## MEDICATION

We have already outlined that some medications unfortunately can cause side effects, which are associated with sexual problems. For example, some antidepressants are associated with difficulties with erections in men. Antiretrovirals are associated with a host of different side effects. Some of these, such as neuropathy may be involved in causing sexual problems such as erectile dysfunction because it affects the nervous system.

## ALCOHOL AND DRUGS

These can clearly affect your body and have a major effect on sexual response. The types of substance and the amount that is taken will have different effects on different people. Some people may take to drinking alcohol more to cope with their HIV related problems. Unfortunately this may add to problems rather than help. For example, it could impair your sexual functioning through loss of erections, general disinhibition, or there may be difficulties in finding a partner due to alcohol-related unsociable behaviour, such as aggression. If this applies to you, you may like to review your alcohol or substance intake to enable you to have more satisfying sexual experiences.

# 2. PSYCHOLOGICAL

People often view sex as a physical activity and therefore might regard biological factors as the most important in sexual problems. In fact, psychological factors can affect sexual functioning just as dramatically. In people under the age of 40 years they are the most common reasons for sexual problems. Sometimes, there may be physical and psychological factors operating together that need to be considered. If a sexual problem occurs only in specific sexual situations rather than generally, it is more likely to be caused by psychological factors.

For example, if a man finds that he can obtain erections with casual partners and with solo masturbation, but not with regular partners, it shows the mechanics are working fine and suggest a difficulty with, for example, intimacy. If psychological problems could be the cause for your sexual problems, it might be helpful to explore the possibility of psychotherapy or counselling to find out what the psychological cause of these problems could be and what might be done to address them.

## LIFE EVENTS

A wide range of life events (unemployment, relationship loss, excessive work demands, illness etc.) may trigger psychological reactions, such as stress and depression. These are very difficult emotional states to cope with and while people are suffering from these they frequently experience sexual problems. These are often related to reduced sexual desire. If this is the case for you psychotherapy or counselling might be helpful.

## UNSUITABLE CIRCUMSTANCES

Physically and psychologically there are times when sex is just not going to feel good for you. You may feel tired, hurried or preoccupied with other things. Also, you may feel that you lack privacy, warmth or comfort. In relation to having HIV, it might just not be the right time to have sex. For example, if you have come home from the hospital after having found out that your viral load is rising it is very understandable that you might not be in the mood for sex. There may be other circumstances related to your HIV when you might feel like this.

Despite the above, many people attempt sex when exhausted or under the wrong circumstances. As a result they then feel frustrated with themselves if their level of fatigue or other factors interfere with their ability to enjoy sex. It is helpful to develop a more understanding attitude towards yourself and accept that there will not always be the right time for sex. The more understanding and accepting you are with yourself about this, the easier it will also be for your partner to accept this and positively support you. This will release you from a lot of the pressure, which you may have been placing on yourself and will enable you to enjoy those times when it feels really good to have sex.

## YOUR PARTNER'S REACTION TO THE SEXUAL PROBLEM

Sex is mostly interactive, involving two people, who provide each other with stimulation, communication and continuous non-verbal and verbal feedback. The way in which you respond to each other in your relationships will play a key role in the development of sexual problems and whether such difficulties are likely to occur.

In a loving and understanding relationship you may be able to deal with sexual problems much more effectively than in a relationship that places all responsibility for the sexual difficulties on you. Indeed, sexual problems should be seen as belonging to the couple, rather than to you alone. Therefore if you do consider seeking professional help for your sexual problems it would be very helpful if your partner could be included or at least take an interest and actively support you with this.

## GENERAL QUALITY OF THE RELATIONSHIP

Relationship and sexual difficulties are frequently found to coexist. Sexual problems may reflect problems in your relationship. In addition, a problematic sexual relationship may have an adverse effect on your relationship in general. There are many relationship interactions that can affect your sexual relationship. These can include feeling angry, bitter or resentful towards your partner, or feeling insecure or frightened with your partner. In relation to having HIV, they can include feelings of resentment or guilt if you are HIV positive and your partner is negative.

These emotions are human and understandable, but they need to be addressed if they are not to get in the way of you enjoying a good relationship, including your sexual interactions. If you feel that these emotions affect your relationship or sexual interactions it could be very helpful to seek professional support to help you work through these emotions.

## NEGATIVE EMOTIONS

Distressing emotions such as fear, anger, guilt, disgust, and shame can all interfere with your sexual functioning. Mental health problems, such as depression and anxiety, can also cause problems with sexual functioning. People who have been exposed to trauma, including sexual assault or abuse, frequently also report problems with sexual functioning.

Feeling depressed, worthless or not deserving of pleasure will obviously inhibit your sexual enjoyment. Similarly, feeling unattractive and unhappy with your body will have the same effect. In relation to HIV, people report that HIV has affected their self-image, which in a sexual context can have a major adverse affect. If you feel that you are affected by any of the above, it could be very helpful to address these distressing emotions with a professional and find out what you might be able to do to about it.

## BAD FEELINGS ASSOCIATED WITH SEX

There are many general types of 'bad' feelings associated with sex, some of which you may also have experienced. These can include:

- fear of pregnancy or pain
- fear of being 'caught', overheard or interrupted
- fear of performance failure
- fear of losing control (i.e.: becoming animal-like, undignified, incontinent, unattractive)
- feeling guilt (i.e.: believing that sex is wrong)
- feeling disgust (i.e.: feeling that sex is dirty or messy).

In terms of having HIV, people have reported unhelpful feelings, such as fear of infecting a partner; fear of being rejected sexually; or fear of being more unattractive because of HIV, which may cause sexual avoidance. Often these feelings can be challenged by your acceptance of your HIV status and checking out the reality behind some of these fears, such as by dating people.

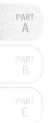

## BELIEFS,
## MISUNDERSTANDING AND LACK OF INFORMATION

Beliefs about sex exert a huge influence over your sexual functioning. We all tend to hold our own beliefs about sexual activities, such as, which sexual activities are acceptable, pleasurable, when, where and with whom. There are also beliefs about sex roles, such as, who can do what, to whom and about what good sex consists of, for example, the role of passion or the importance of spontaneity.

Some beliefs can make you more vulnerable to developing sexual problems than others. For example, if a man holds the belief that the key to good sex is only up to him during penetration, he is more likely to experience performance anxiety. Also, a woman thinking that she can become infected with HIV through kissing will limit what she does and it will impact on her enjoyment. You might find it helpful to read the paragraph, on Myths and Truths about HIV infection during sex in this Chapter to find out more about what is safe and what is not.

## SKILL

It takes practice to put on a condom properly or to feel good about what you do during sex and find out what your partner enjoys. Unlike in the movies sex is not always spontaneous and perfect. Changing your sexual practices to being safer might also require some practice in other ways, such as, for example, deciding to focus more on non-penetrative sex when you are not used to doing this. There are some books that might help you to find out more and experiment with non-penetrative sexual practices.

PART
A

PART
B

PART
C

## COMMUNICATION

Sexual problems often stem from communication problems within the relationship. For example, they may relate to the way in which either partner expresses their needs and desires (or doesn't), a lack of clarity regarding expectations or an inability to communicate boundaries. It is therefore very important to carefully look at the way in which you communicate with your partner, the effect that this has on your relationship and the way in which it may have an affect upon your sexual relationship.

It is never too late to learn new ways of communicating, whether you are in a long-term relationship, short-term relationship or single. Good interpersonal communication is essential for all human interactions, and helps to resolve sexual problems.

Figure (18) on the next page shows five basic principles of interpersonal communication:

**1** Aim to communicate with each other as two adults - notice those situations in which either you or your partner, or both of you move out of a "healthy adult" mode and go into a child-like mode, this can interfere with constructive communication. You can notice this by focussing in on yourself to feel whether you experience yourself as your present day adult or somehow smaller, more vulnerable or weaker. Treat each other with dignity and respect. Remember to treat your partner in the way in which you would also like to be treated.

**2** Teach yourself to 'self-assert' and 'self-protect'– in other words being in touch with your needs. Learn to state your needs clearly, but be prepared also to listen to the needs of others. Improve your personal boundaries and become aware how much of your energy or resources you can give to the other and at what point you will have to stop. Learn to communicate this clearly, firmly and kindly. If you are upset with the other person try to explain how the other person is affecting you and what your needs are rather than being critical and angry.

**3** Remember that you are entitled to your own feelings and you should be allowed to express these freely - likewise respect that your partner is equally entitled to the same rights. However, expressing your feelings should not put your partner in the position to become your rescuer or to solve problems for you. Expressing your feelings enables you to own them and know that they are a part of you at that point in time.

**4** Keep negotiating what you want, especially on occasions when you want something different - negotiate in a constructive manner, making positive requests rather than

**Fig. 18** Common communication principles

PART
A

PART
B

PART
C

being demanding or manipulative with your partner. However, also remember that being in a partnership usually involves some form of compromise. Aim to negotiate win-win situations between yourself and your partner.

**5** Use praise and encouragement. Work hard at noticing and commenting on the good things, which your partner does - the more positives you bring into your relationship, the more likely it is that your partner will aim to move to do the same. Essentially, it is very nice to make the other feel valued and appreciated.

PART
A

PART
B

PART
C

SELF-MONITORING: A CHANCE TO CHECK-IN WITH YOURSELF * *sexual problems* ( I ) *Looking at the many physical and psychological causes of sexual problems, do any affect you? (2) Have you solutions to remedy any sexual problems you may have? What are they? Have you tried them? It could be very helpful to make some notes about the above in your diary, notebook or on a sheet of paper, so that you can later decide on what might help you to take some of your observations further.*

# DISCLOSURE AND SEXUAL RELATIONSHIPS

Disclosure of HIV status to a sexual partner has often been confused with responsibility and safer sex. Safer sex does not always require disclosure of HIV status. It is perfectly possible to have good sex where there is no risk of transmission without ever mentioning HIV, for example, with mutual masturbation.

Disclosure is ideally of your choice and in your control. Nevertheless, disclosure is an important and often tricky issue that comes up for people with HIV who live in relationships. At times it may feel like there is undue and unfair pressure placed on you to disclose. This can leave you feeling guilty about non-disclosure before you have been able to ask yourself whether you feel safe and comfortable enough to disclose. It is not possible to prescribe one approach to the issue. However, it could be very helpful for you to have a framework within which to think about disclosure issues. Only you can decide on what is really best for you and it is important that you stay within your own integrity, whatever your decision. Chapter 4 discusses the issue of disclosure in more detail.

PART
A

PART
B

PART
C

# CONCLUSION

Many people living with HIV experience satisfying intimate relationships and sexual lives. While it is true that the medical and psychological aspects of HIV infection can make it harder to achieve this, this is not necessarily the case. There are, for instance, people who report much more satisfying sexual relationships post diagnosis. It is therefore very possible for you to enjoy good and safe sex, despite being HIV positive.

When problems occur, whether they are about desire, arousal, orgasm, or with general communication, there are effective therapies for sexual problems. These can be physical (e.g. Viagra), psychological (psychotherapy or counselling) or a combination of both. Also they can take place individually or as a couple. Most HIV clinics should have referral pathways for such problems and to professionals (such as Clinical Psychologists) that can treat sexual problems and see people on their own or with their partner.

# Child and Family HIV

# INTRODUCTION

HIV can affect anyone and over the past ten years, there has been an increase in the numbers of HIV infected children. As people are living longer on medication, it is not just adults who are HIV positive, but also babies, children and adolescents.

Having a family of your own may be one of your main wishes in life. For some people it may be an important personal goal or an expected family goal due to the culture they come from. Whilst starting a family carries with it many new responsibilities in itself, having HIV creates additional considerations that we will look at in this chapter.

Babies, children and adolescents also have specific issues that arise for them if they are HIV positive or have HIV positive parents, which we will describe.

This chapter offers an overview of the key issues in relation to pregnancy, children and family life for people negotiating life with HIV.

# DECIDING TO HAVE A CHILD

Despite being HIV positive you can still have many of the same choices open to you now as you did prior to being diagnosed HIV positive. This includes the decision about having a child. However, if you choose to have children or achieve pregnancy you will need to take into account your own health status, your partner's health status and the health of the unborn baby.

There are different sero-status combinations that can occur with HIV positive couples or individuals who want a child. The following lists some possible relationship combinations and each will have its own HIV-related issues. Are any of these combinations relevant to your own situation?

- When both partners are HIV positive (sero-concordance)
- When one partner is HIV positive and one HIV negative (sero-discordance)
- When one partner is HIV positive, but the status of the other partner is not known
- When neither partner knows their HIV status

The above scenarios and their specific HIV-related issues need to be carefully considered. If any of these combinations apply to you and you want to start a family or have another child it would be important to discuss your intentions with and seek the advice of an appropriate medical professional. It is not uncommon for sero-discordant couples (when one is HIV positive and the other HIV negative), now that people are living longer and trying to have as normal a life as possible, to consider the possibility of having children. Developments in obstetrics, paediatrics and HIV services allow for more lifestyle choices for people with HIV, such as the possibility of having a child. "Sperm washing" might be considered and practised, where the male partner is HIV positive.

**What is Sperm Washing?** *Sperm washing sounds quite strange, but it is actually a unique technological development in the reduction of HIV transmission. Sperm washing is the process of reducing HIV transmission from the sperm to the woman. The sperm from the HIV positive man is 'spun' to separate the sperm from the seminal fluid. It is believed that HIV is present in the seminal fluid rather than in the sperm itself. Therefore it is consid-*

PART
A

PART
B

PART
C

*ered safer to use the separated sperm. The couple must agree not to have unprotected sex before and during this time. Sperm washing is not widely available in this country and does have a cost. Discuss this issue with your HIV doctor if you are interested, who can help you think about what options are available for you.*

Bringing a child into this world is a major responsibility that cannot be underestimated, whether you are HIV positive or not. Whether it is the right thing to do for you will depend on your own personal circumstances. Figure (19) shows a decision-making sheet, in which you can start to think about the reasons for and against having a baby. Try filling it out if you are considering having a child. What reasons can you think of 'for' having a child or and what are your reasons 'against' this decision? Examples of reasons 'for' could be: that you are in a stable relationship and have been for some time; you have one child and had

PART
A

PART
B

PART
C

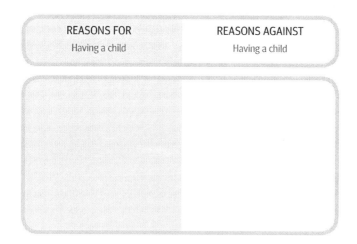

**Fig. 19**  Decision making working out the pros and cose of having a child

no problems and wish to have another; your HIV is well controlled and you have adhered well to the treatment. Examples of reasons 'against' could be that you are not yet adjusted to your own HIV diagnosis and do not feel emotionally ready to have a child; that you feel the relationship that you are in is not working and particular relationship issues need addressing; that you want a child to meet your own needs and are not thinking about the future of the child; that you find it difficult enough to deal with the responsibility of achieving good medication adherence that you are not sure whether you have enough spare energy for dealing with the multiple needs of a baby and child. Whatever your own reasons, they are very important for you to explore and to be aware of. Also they will differ between different people and, probably even between yourself and the partner you are considering having a child with. Therefore it would be very helpful for both of you to complete your own decision sheet separately and later compare and explore the communalities and the differences. Whatever your decision, taking on the responsibility of having a family or another child is a major decision, which cannot be reversed once put into action.

Being able to feel that you have explored the issues carefully and responsibly will help you immensely. If you decide that you really do want to have a child and you are satisfied that your reasons for this are sound, then your sense of clarity can help you feel more at peace with your decision and also during your pregnancy.

PART A

PART B

PART C

## ANTE-NATAL HIV TESTING

Antenatal care is also called prenatal care. Antenatal is the period before a baby's birth, during which the foetus (developing baby) develops and grows in the uterus. A pregnant HIV positive woman can pass on HIV to her baby during pregnancy, labour, delivery and breast-feeding. The numbers of HIV positive children born to African parents is considerably higher than for the rest of the world. This, however, can be prevented if you know that you are HIV positive and take effective and safe methods to reduce the chances of passing on HIV to your baby. If you are thinking of having children now or in the future, it is important to consider having an HIV test for this reason if you currently do not know your status. Antenatal HIV testing is now becoming a routine part of the initial prenatal screening and care.

Whenever you have an HIV test, you will need to consider the range of issues outlined in the chapter on HIV diagnosis (Chapter 1). An HIV diagnosis at any time is difficult for most people. However when you are attempting to start a family or have more children and you are then finding out that you are HIV positive, this can be especially difficult. It may take you considerable time to adjust to this finding. However, you may already be pregnant and therefore it will not just be your own feelings, but also the needs of the baby and your relationship as a couple that you need to take into account.

The following issues will require your consideration at the antenatal stage, if HIV has been diagnosed:

- What effect will an HIV diagnosis have on your relationship as a couple?
- How will HIV change your plans as a couple together?
- How will pregnancy be experienced and what could be the possible complications?
- What HIV treatments and procedures will be required to prevent vertical transmission of HIV from mother to baby?

- Will delivery be planned and how? Will the birth be natural (vaginal) or a Caesarean section (assisted)?
- What formula milks are available to substitute breast milk?
- What other issues after birth (post-natal) need consideration?
- What support will I have with the baby?

The following description of Janet and Marcus' story outlines some common preliminary issues.

*Janet + Marcus* *have been in a relationship for three years. The relationship is very loving and both enjoy the prospect of their future together. They both decided after much thought to have a baby together. Whilst visiting her G.P. for routine gynaecological advice, Janet discussed the issue of wanting to have a child. Her G.P. suggested a HIV test for both Janet and Marcus. Janet suddenly realised that their dream was becoming a source of stress because of the possible implications of being HIV positive. When Janet later met Marcus, she felt overwhelmed by the issue of HIV and felt that it was ruining their chances of happiness as a family. She couldn't talk to Marcus about HIV as she felt that he would be angry with her and they would both experience conflict over the issue.*

PART
A

PART
B

PART
C

What can Janet and Marcus do in this situation? Should the prospect of HIV testing and the possibility of an HIV test realistically ruin the chances of starting a family with a child? The answers are clearly individual and once the possibility of HIV comes into the picture additional implications arise, which previously would not have occurred as an issue to most couples.

# PREGNANCY AND DELIVERY
## SOME IMPORTANT FACTS

☛ **How is HIV transmitted to a baby?** *(1) Without HIV treatment, about 25% of babies born to HIV+ women will be born HIV+. (2) The exact way that transmission from mother to baby happens is still unknown. However the majority of transmissions occur near the time of or during labour and delivery when the baby is being born. It can also occur through breast-feeding (3) Certain risk factors can make transmission during birth more probable. One main risk factor is the mother's viral load; another is the time between the mother's water breaking and the actual delivery.*

☛ **How do HIV drugs protect the baby?** *(1) The risk of your baby becoming HIV+ can be reduced with anti-HIV therapy. (2) An American and French joint study (trial) showed that mothers who took the anti-HIV drug AZT before and during labour and where the baby received AZT for six weeks after birth reduced the risk of the baby becoming infected from 25% to 8%. (3) From 1994, this strategy has been recommended for all HIV+ women. Since then further advances in treatment have reduced transmission rates with a planned birth and combination therapy to less than 1%. (3) Each mother will need to discuss the benefits and the risks of this treatment with both paediatric and adult HIV services. In some hospitals there are close links between the adult HIV Physician and the Paediatricians.*

Good health and a low viral load are very important if you are thinking of having children. The healthier you are, the better chance your baby has of being healthy, too. The chapter on Healthy Lifestyles in this book will

156

be relevant to maintaining your health whilst being HIV positive. Specific gynaecological issues for women also may need addressing, such as:

- regular cervical smear tests
- contraceptive advice
- counselling and referral for termination of pregnancy, if appropriate
- breast examinations
- management of menstruation problems
- infertility problems, and so on

It is important that you look after yourself and agree to medical monitoring and help with any of the above issues as they become relevant. Your local Family Planning Services can help with these issues.

PART A

PART B

PART C

SELF-MONITORING: A CHANCE TO CHECK-IN WITH YOURSELF • *Having a child* ( 1 ) *Before being diagnosed HIV positive did you ever want to have children? Is having a child a major life goal for you? (2) Since your diagnosis have your wishes for having a child changed? Why? In what way? What problems do you see with it now that you are HIV positive? It could be very helpful to make some notes about the above in your diary, notebook or on a sheet of paper, so that you can later decide on what might help you to take some of your observations further.*

## BREAST FEEDING

*Tanya* is HIV positive and lives with her HIV positive partner, John. She has just given birth by Caesarean section to a *beautiful baby boy, called Jacob. Tanya instinctually feels the need to breastfeed, but after discussing the issue of breast milk and HIV transmission with her doctors and other staff, she has agreed with her partner to use formula milk instead. Whilst at a routine postnatal check-up in a non-HIV clinic, Tanya sees posters stating that 'Breast is Best'. She is overwhelmed with sadness and feels guilty, ashamed and a bad mother to Jacob for not being able to breastfeed him. Tanya just wants to do what she thought all mothers did and breastfeed. To add to her distress, another mother at the clinic sits next to her and starts breastfeeding her own new baby. The other mother describes with pride to Tanya that breast-feeding is a wonderful and special experience. She turns to Tanya and asks how she is experiencing her own breastfeeding.*

When you have HIV it is essential that you do not breastfeed your child under any circumstances, as this can cause transmission of the virus. However, not being able to breastfeed can cause many issues for a mother, as can be seen in Tanya's case, above. Many mothers find it very difficult not to breastfeed for the first few days after their baby's birth, especially, when their milk starts to come in. Breastfeeding is such a natural instinct and if you have given birth to a lovely baby, it can be emotionally very painful to have to resist your natural instinct of wanting to breastfeed your newborn baby.

Another difficulty you will have to cope with is the initial physical discomfort, as your breasts are full and you are not able to give this milk to your baby. It can feel very difficult to have to extract your milk to ease your discomfort and not give this milk to your baby. However, despite these very natural instincts and urges in you and the resulting difficult emotional and physical sensations, it is important that you do not breastfeed your baby. This will help your baby's protection from HIV.

Sometimes mothers can be very worried that being seen to be bottle-feeding will identify them as HIV positive. It is up to you whether or not you tell anyone that you are HIV positive. There can also be significant social pressure about not being seen to be breastfeeding, as the example about Tanya demonstrates. It can be very difficult to be confronted by other mothers who are breastfeeding and you may feel guilty or depressed about not being able to do the same for your baby. If you find yourself in such situations, remember that you are doing the best for your baby, you are protecting it and you are taking responsibility for your baby's future health. Whatever others may think or say, it is important that you are very clear yourself what you do and why you are doing this for your baby.

If you do not wish to tell anyone that you are not breast-feeding because you are HIV positive, your doctor or midwife will be able to help you with reasons to explain why you are not breast-feeding. There can be many other reasons for why a woman does not breastfeed her baby, such as having cracked nipples; that there wasn't enough milk; that the baby developed colic after the breast milk or others. However, what will be important when you can't breastfeed your baby that you give your baby just as much closeness, warmth and attention as you would naturally have to do with breastfeeding, when you are bottle-feeding. Research in neurobiology has shown that affectionate bonding is best achieved if you place your baby on your left arm as you are bottle-feeding, so that your baby's left ear is free and facing you. You can then comfort your baby by singing to your baby or whispering loving words while feeding. It is important that you maintain loving eye contact with your baby as you are doing this.

PART
A

PART
B

PART
C

# PAEDIATRIC HIV

Unfortunately, sometimes babies are born HIV+, when the mother doesn't know her own diagnosis or comes from a country where treatment was not available. All babies and children, who are HIV+ in the UK, will be designated to a Paediatrician at a Paediatric HIV treatment centre, or a Paediatrician attached to a local HIV paediatric team. This doctor will be central in the HIV monitoring process. Other professional staff may also be needed, such as Nurses, Clinical Psychologists, Dieticians, Social Workers and potential others.

As a parent, you know your child better than anyone else. If you notice any symptoms or have any worries about anything you observe in your child it will be important that you report this to your Paediatrician. If your child is infected with HIV there are several reasons to attend regularly for check-ups. For example, to find out if any problems are developing, for reassurance about your child's progress and to ask questions about anything you are uncertain of. It is important and your responsibility to keep regular clinic appointments. The frequency of these may vary, depending on the age of your child, how well he or she is and what treatments are required. Your Paediatrician and the associated healthcare team will explain to you what is needed for enabling a good monitoring of your child's needs so that you know what to expect. If all is well, appointments will often be just routine check-ups.

# PREPARING YOUR CHILD FOR A HOSPITAL VISIT

Hospitals can often be scary places for children. Preparing your child beforehand through talking, reading and playing can help your child understand and feel more relaxed about the clinic visits. Distracting your child with music, books or toys during painful procedures may help your child feel less overwhelmed and affected by the procedures. Remaining calm and relaxed and not showing your distress to your child will also help. While you do not want to overwhelm your child with your own distress, it could be very helpful if you had an outlet for your distress elsewhere. If your child is affected by HIV and if there are issues that really upset you, it could be helpful if you sought some independent professional support, such as psychotherapy or counselling for yourself.

Other children in the family may also need to be prepared and reassured as they, too, can become frightened and upset as they may experience their sibling going through more examinations and check-ups compared to themselves. They may also feel resentful, as they might feel left out because their sibling seems to be getting more attention. It is important to try and include all the children equally and allow special times also for the children who do not have special healthcare requirements. It is also very important to ensure that the affected child feels included within the family and, depending on their developmental age and the child's level of understanding, feels part of the issues the family faces.

PART
A

PART
B

PART
C

# CAN A CHILD PASS ON HIV TO OTHERS?

Parents and carers may worry that their child with HIV could infect another child. There is no evidence that children can pass on HIV during everyday activities. As a basic rule, everyone should be encouraged to wash their hands with soap and water and dry them before preparing food and after any activity where germs may be present. This is especially important, as a HIV infected child may be more vulnerable to other's germs.

Any situation where blood is drawn, such as a scratch from a fall, is where extra care should be taken. After cleaning wounds with soap and water, cover sores, cuts, grazes with a waterproof plaster for 24-hours, or until a scab has formed. Keep covered if the wound weeps or bleeds again. If blood splashes into eyes, mouth or on skin, wash immediately with cold water. If blood is spilt, mop it up with a disposable tissue or towel. Ultimately, always use the most logical and hygienic method.

**Should the school that my child is attending know that my child is HIV+?** *Schools do not have to be told of your child's HIV positive diagnosis. All schools should have been given advice from the Department of Health around standards and procedures for dealing with accidents. There should also be protocols for general hygiene. If you chose to tell the Head Teacher or Class Teacher they may be able to offer you some understanding and support if your child has to miss school due to hospital appointments or illness or needs to take medication at school. It is ultimately your choice, but should only be done if it helps to support your child.*

# DISCLOSURE – WHEN AND HOW?

You will need to decide when it is the most appropriate time to tell your children of their HIV diagnosis and yours. If you have other children who do not have HIV you may feel that they also should know. Deciding when and how to tell is not easy but it is also not easy keeping secrets.

## DISCLOSING AN HIV DIAGNOSIS TO A CHILD

DISCLOSURE will depend on the child's mental ability, maturity, age and understanding. The best time to start the disclosure process is between the ages of 9-13 years. Each situation will be different and circumstances vary for each child. The most important aspect is that whenever you decide that it is the right time to disclose that you use a developmentally appropriate approach to do so.

DISCLOSURE should occur in small stages and it can take several years before partial to full disclosure has occurred. Partial disclosure could be that you explain hospital visits as a way to check that the child's blood is OK and that some children have to do this. What to say can be thought about and implemented with the help of professionals, such as your Paediatrician or a Clinical Child Psychologist.

DISCLOSURE must remain an ongoing, open and honest dialogue. Your child may need time to get used to ideas or procedures and as this happens, new issues and questions may arise. Talking and listening must occur throughout this process so that feelings can be expressed and processed in a child-appropriate manner. It is important that you maintain the truth at all times, but explain things in a way that your child can understand.

DISCLOSURE Enables your child to understand and participate in their own healthcare and other important decisions, especially in preparation for the time when they may increasingly negotiate their own health care for themselves as adolescents. Knowledge and control are important factors in helping reduce stress and distress.

PART A

PART B

PART C

Fig. 20  Disclosing HIV to a child

Keeping secrets in this case is not the best solution. Children are very perceptive and sensitive and they can often pick up on parents' conversations, moods and worries.

Every family is different and there is no set age at which to tell, but you can start to gently prepare your child or children by helping them to learn gradually about HIV in understandable terms. In this context it is very important to provide honest answers to children's questions, but in a manner that takes into consideration the child's level of development and understanding. Conversations with children need to occur in an age appropriate manner without burdening your child unnecessarily with responsibilities, which they are not ready to carry, yet. At the same time, it can be very helpful if your child can learn to appreciate that some personal information, such as being HIV positive, should be dealt with sensitively and not everybody will respond to your child in an understanding and supportive manner. Therefore you might plan together with your child, who the specific people are that your child might be able to talk to about their condition and who your child should not talk to about their HIV status.

## ADOLESCENT TRANSITIONAL ISSUES

There are now children with HIV who have reached their adolescence. For all children adolescence is an emotionally very difficult transitional time, which frequently brings up a lot of issues. For children with an HIV diagnosis, moving into adolescence can even be more challenging and good support for them will be needed. The following list highlights some key issues that can arise in adolescence, including some additional issues relating to having HIV. Frequently, enabling your children to have a safe space to talk in or people to talk to who they feel particularly close to can help them to deal with some of these issues better. This may be members within the family, friends or professionals, who they have developed particular trust in over the years.

- CONTROL AND AUTONOMY - for example, exploring personal boundaries, which issues the adolescent can, take control of and which not; understanding when autonomy might be encouraged and where the adolescent may assume autonomy before they have reached sufficient emotional maturity.
- IDENTITY AND SELF ESTEEM – for example, questions about the purpose of being in this world; for the adolescent to develop a sense of their particular strengths, talents and those aspects that make them unique; developing and feeling a sense of worth as a person.
- PHYSICAL AND PERSONALITY DEVELOPMENTS – for example, the need to explore their body, their bodily changes and their emerging sexuality; having a sense of their preferences and dislikes.
- RELATIONSHIPS: FRIENDSHIPS/PEER AND INTIMATE/SEXUAL – for example, defining themselves in terms of who their peers are and who not; starting to develop sexual interests and sexual relationships.
- FEELING DIFFERENT AND ISOLATED FROM PEERS AND MANAGING SECRECY – for example, not being able to tell friends about their HIV status; feeling alone with having to go to check-ups when friends would not have to think about issues like that; feeling resentful about not being able to engage in sexuality as freely and innocently as their friends might.
- COPING WITH ACADEMIC PRESSURES AND EXAMINATIONS AND FUTURE CAREER PLANNING – for example, thinking more about particular interests and talents and finding the right courses at school to

support these; fear in adolescents with HIV that their future career might look different compared to that of their friends; anxiety about having less time and less opportunities than friends; feeling that own priorities are quite different compared to those of friends.

- ADHERENCE TO HIV MEDICATIONS WITH INCREASING SELF-RESPONSIBILITY – for example, realization that adherence to HIV medication will have to be life-long and ongoing; increased understanding and coping with HIV related issues; less involvement of parents or carers in adolescent's decision regarding their HIV medication and other life choices.
- TRANSFER FROM PAEDIATRIC HIV SERVICES TO ADULT HIV SERVICES – for example, adjusting to a different level of support and care and a different set of Professionals.

# FAMILIES LIVING WITH HIV

Healthy relationships and positive attachment styles within the family are vital for a child to deal with having HIV. Feeling safe, secure, loved and nurtured in a consistent manner will buffer a child's experience of having HIV. A cohesive family can achieve many things together – no matter how many people exist within the family framework. It is always important to consider how HIV affects particular members of the family and also during each new phase of a child's life. Sometimes this may feel difficult as you may be trying to cope with your own problems or concerns, while at the same time trying to protect another family member, such as your children, from your own worries. It is often helpful to have some outside support, whether this is a partner, friend or a professional who you trust and with whom you can be totally open about your concerns.

It is important also to remember the needs of affected children, who might not necessarily have HIV themselves, but have parents or siblings, who do. The example of Anna, below, illustrates some of the issues an affected child might have, such as fears and questions about HIV in relation to themselves, members of their family and their futures.

*Anna* *is 8 years old and HIV negative. She is the youngest of three children. Her older brothers are ten and fourteen years old. Both are HIV positive and have been since birth. Anna has overheard some heated discussions between her mother and her brothers and words and names are being used, such as 'HIV' and 'Hospital' and 'Anna'. This has made Anna feel scared that something bad might happen to someone, possibly to her. She has begun to withdraw when at home and she has stopped being her usual bright self. Her mother has noticed this change and has asked Anna what the problem is. Anna reluctantly explained her fears and her mother realised that now may be the right time to start the process of disclosure. With time Anna learned to appreciate that her brothers are needing to go through their own adjustment process and that she started to feel much more settled and happier again.*

PART A

PART B

PART C

### SELF-MONITORING: A CHANCE TO CHECK-IN WITH YOURSELF ∗ *who is in your family* ( / ) *How many people make up your immediate and extended family? Who are you most close to, what roles do members in your family have? How do you see yourself in relation to your family? How do you think your family see you? Are there other family members who are HIV+? (2) Who*

*in your family knows about your HIV status? If so, why did you tell them? What have you learned from telling? If you have close family members, who are 'affected', what do you think their experience of HIV is? It could be very helpful to make some notes about the above in your diary, notebook or on a sheet of paper, so that you can later decide on what might help you to take some of your observations further.*

You may like to allow yourself to think about who is in your family and what their issues are in relation to HIV. You might like to consider some of the questions, below, to explore the individual and communal needs of particular members of your family in relation to HIV.

# THINKING ABOUT FAMILY RELATIONSHIPS AND HIV

- What are relationships like in your family - close or distant?
- Who knows about HIV in your family?
- What is the level of understanding of HIV in your family?
- How do your family members cope with HIV?
- How do problems affect your family members?
- How would you know if your child was not coping with having HIV?
- What could you do to help your child if this was the case?
- If problems occur for the family how would the family resolve them?
- Do you know how other people deal with the same issues?
- What solutions and resources are available within your family?
- Which other people are or might need to be included so that your family experiences sufficient support in coping with the HIV?

# CONCLUSION

Having HIV will mean that there will have to be certain changes in your life. However, it does not necessarily mean a dramatic change to everyday life. You and your family can carry on doing the same things you have been doing or would like to do. There is, for example, no reason why you can't have a child, your child cannot start playgroup or school, or stay at a friend's house or participate in sports' activities (including swimming). There is no reason why you should not be able to experience love, happiness and joy towards each other in your family. In some ways, HIV may be the impetus for allowing you to live your life more consciously and more fully. It may have made you become more aware of what the really important issues in your life are and the ones, which are more peripheral. You may also experience more closeness and warmth rather than less, because you may have a different sense of how precious and, yet, vulnerable life and human existence really is.

The psychological well being of your family and all the members within it is important for all concerned in order to be able to cope with the many issues HIV will throw up, in whatever circumstances you may find yourself in. The more you allow yourself to be understanding and compassionate of your own and other peoples' issues the better you will be able to deal with them.

PART
A

PART
B

PART
C

# 7

# Understanding
# HIV–Associated Emotions

# INTRODUCTION

We all experience emotions every day of our lives. If you are living with HIV infection you will experience many emotions associated with it and sometimes these emotions can be difficult to cope with.

This chapter will explain the nature of emotions, outline the importance and usefulness of emotions and explain common emotions associated with HIV infection.

# WHAT ARE EMOTIONS?

The ability to feel emotions is what defines us as human beings. Emotions consist of a mixture of feelings and bodily sensations, which can be triggered in response to a wide variety of situations or factors. In order to explain in more detail how and why emotional reactions are triggered we will use the following example: Imagine a situation where a friend, who you hadn't seen sneaking up on you, suddenly jumps up at you from behind, surprising you.

When you are surprised, your brain quickly appraises the situation. It has to decide whether it is an unknown situation or whether you may have been in similar circumstances before, whether the situation could represent a threat, in which case it has to prepare you to act, or whether this is a pleasant situation and you can relax. This evaluation takes place very speedily and your whole nervous system, including your brain is equipped to scan and evaluate new situations on many levels.

In the situation where your friend suddenly jumps at you from behind, you may feel a surprise effect and calm down quickly again. However, in a different situation, which is assessed and registered as

PART
A

PART
B

PART
C

being stressful or even dangerous, your brain handles the immediate response. It does so by signalling the adrenal medulla (part of the adrenal gland), which in response releases two neurotransmitters (our body's own chemicals that carry messages to and from the nerves). These are adrenaline (also called: epinephrine) and noradrenaline (also called: norepinephrine), which are released into the blood by the medullary cells.

The release of these neurotransmitters leads to an increased heart rate, blood pressure and lung function; a constriction of the blood vessels in many parts of the body, but dilation of blood vessels in the muscular system; inhibition of the stomach and intestinal action; dilation of the pupil and inhibition in salivation; relaxation of the bladder and increased metabolism and alertness.

These changes in our body enable us to engage in three potential emergency responses, the "3 'F's", which are all designed to optimize our survival. The first is the "fight" response. This might involve actual fight, or more often, some other way of confronting the dangerous situation. The second is the "flight" response, which enables us to get away from a critical situation. During critical situations, during which neither fight nor flight are possible, a third response is activated (in response to the release of additional chemical compounds). This is referred to as the "freeze" response and this is the most critical of all bodily responses, as it carries enormous costs for the human organism. During the "freeze" response a person goes into a state of numbness (sometimes dissociation), during which they may feel internally quite alert, but are body shuts down and feels immobilized. This state can also be observed in mammals, when predators chase them and they literally freeze or loose all muscle tone and flop down, so that the predator might mistake them for dead. This state is often associated with severe stress, such as traumatic experiences that can lead to posttraumatic stress disorder. After an acute episode of stress, cortisol, a hormone produced in the adrenal cortex (part of the adrenal gland) is released in order to restore the body back to homeostasis.

While the emergency measure of the stress response is vital under certain situations, it can also be disruptive and damaging, especially if it is triggered in situations, which don't require one of those 3 emergency responses. For example, we may find our "fight" response activated in situations, where physical action is inappropriate, dangerous or even illegal and under these circumstances activation of the stress response can take a significant toll on our body and mind. In situations of prolonged and chronic stress, prolonged cortisol secretion has been found, which not only changes the natural patterns of serum cortisol in the body, but also leads to the negative long-term effects of stress on our physical and mental well being, as mentioned, above.

# EIGHT PRIMARY HUMAN EMOTIONS

There are eight primary human emotions that are thought to have a biological or innate basis: happiness, fear, sadness, anger, disgust, shame, surprise, and interest. There are other emotions known as secondary emotions that are learnt and are usually combinations of these primary emotions. These we will discuss later. First lets look at the eight primary emotions.

- Happiness
- Fear

- Sadness
- Anger
- Disgust
- Shame
- Surprise
- Interest

SELF-MONITORING: A CHANCE TO CHECK-IN WITH YOURSELF • *primary emotions* (1) *Firstly, can you think of times when you experienced the eight primary emotions? Can you think about what they were like in your body, what you thought about them, how they felt, and how they made you react? What were the situations that they occurred in? Were they useful to you? (2) Secondly, were these emotions reactions to events or did they influence events? It could be very helpful to write these down in your diary, notebook or on a sheet of paper, so that you can later decide on what might help you to tackle some of these.*

PART
A

PART
B

PART
C

# EMOTIONS ARE REACTIONS TO EVENTS

Emotions can be either reactions to events in the environment (e.g. receiving a gift, someone being rude) or reactions to thoughts, emotions and behaviour. Certain types of emotion tend to be associated with certain type of events. For example, feeling a sense of happiness can be associated with being paid a compliment, receiving a gift, meeting someone close to you, pleasure through sexual activity, feeling loved by another person and so on.

# EMOTIONS INFLUENCE EVENTS

Emotions have strong effects on the way you think and behave. This can sometimes influence how you react to subsequent events so that the same emotion grows in strength. This is often what people mean when they say "I was already in a bad mood", when they are explaining the way they reacted to an event. For example, if you are on your way to work and discover the telephone company has not done what it promised in fixing your phone line. You may be feeling angry. On arrival to work, you discover that a meeting has been cancelled and you were not told. You are likely to feel even angrier now compared to the time when the only negative thing was the event with the telephone company. Similarly, if you were just diagnosed HIV positive you may feel a whole range of negative emotions. However, with time, you may come to realize that not only do you have to cope with the emotions relating to your diagnosis, but you also have to face and keep adjusting to, a whole range of issues, which will arise in your life. This is likely to affect your mood.

Frequently, our emotions influence the way, in which we are thinking about things, how we perceive things to be, both in the here-and-now and in the past, and how we subsequently behave. This can happen without there being another event to keep them going. They can cause a kind of emotional hangover. When you have experienced sadness you may think about other times when you were sad or lost things and you may focus on all the sad things that you perceive happening around you and find it much harder to think about positive things. This will keep your feelings of sadness alive. Similarly, when you have experienced happiness, you may think about other happy times and your focus may be more on the happy things in your environment.

PART
A

PART
B

PART
C

# THE COMPONENTS
# AND PROPERTIES OF EMOTIONS

In summary, emotions contain the following components:

- Interpretation of events
- Changes to brain chemistry, through the release
  of particular neurotransmitters
- Facial and body changes
- Urges to act
- Behaviour

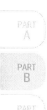

Emotions also have the following properties:

- Certain types of emotions will be associated
  with similar types of events
- They have strong effects on your thinking, body and behaviour
- They can be self-perpetuating

# WHAT USES DO EMOTIONS HAVE?

You will have experienced times when you wished that your emotions did not exist, because they were intense and difficult to cope with. Emotions, however, are an integral part of being a human. They are very important and vital sources of information and wisdom. In fact, humans could not survive and function without them. Emotions are part of your internal communication system, which exists to let you know when things feel good and when not and they guide you to take appropriate action, sometimes at the level of ensuring your very own survival. The following example gives a snapshot of what it would be to live without emotions.

*Chris wakes up one morning and the sun is shining. Because happiness does not exist this makes no difference. He goes for a walk in the park and bumps into a friend who he has not seen for a long time. As surprise does not exist, the meeting is not appreciated and Chris perceives no feelings while in conversation with his friend. He then goes to a shop and the shop attendant is rude to him. As anger does not exist he does not notice that he is treated badly and receives an unhelpful service. Finally, while crossing the road he notices a car speeding towards him. As fear does not exist, he fails to move out of the way in time.*

Life would not only be pretty meaningless without emotions, but actually threatening to our survival. Mankind would be reduced to leading a robot-like existence. Furthermore, emotions can be great motivators. For example, throughout history, emotions have motivated people to stand up for their own values to try and create change.

# EMOTIONS ARE ADAPTIVE

Emotions adapt to signals in your external and internal environment and fulfil a range of uses for you. They can do the following:

- Communicate to you about your surroundings, as well as, your own internal situation. They are signs that something

PART
A

PART
B

PART
C

has or is happening. They communicate to you what
is important to you in your life (and what is not)

- Help you communicate to others how you feel
- Motivate you to do things you would not otherwise do
- Prepare you to act, which is especially vital in situations of emergency
- Help you to act "automatically", therefore saving time in critical situations without you having to think everything through.

# COMMON EMOTIONS ASSOCIATED WITH HIV INFECTION

You may have experienced many emotions triggered by having HIV. These emotions can, in turn, reinforce your experiences of HIV. They can vary in their intensity and frequency. Most people find that their emotions will become stronger in intensity and frequency after diagnosis. Understandably, you have suddenly been given information that has life-altering consequences for you. For most people this is an extremely emotional period in their lives, which can feel very uncomfortable and painful. You need time to adjust to this information and to come to terms with your emotional reactions. The task will eventually be for you to learn to recognize and understand your feelings, accept them and carry on with living the life you want regardless.

## FEAR

Everyone experiences fear from time to time and it is one of the most common emotions that people living with HIV experience. There are many ways in which HIV can represent a threat or danger to you.

A few examples are given below:

- Threat to your health and life
- Threat of rejection by others
- Threat to your identity
- Threat to your self-esteem

There are many uncertainties associated with HIV infection and it is not surprising therefore that you may experience fear around what the future may hold for you. In addition, the degree of uncertainty you may experience tends to increase when there are changes taking place, such as with the readjustments you may need to make as a result of being HIV positive.

You may experience fear in relation to decisions around changing medication. This is because, amongst other things, you may be uncertain about side effects and the effectiveness of the drugs. You may experience fear around disclosure, because you believe it may lead to rejection by others. Sometimes this fear is so great that you might avoid meeting others. Fear can also be experienced when you lose a sense of control over your environment, believing yourself to be helpless. This arises for most people living with HIV infection at some stage.

The challenge will be for you to recognize that you are experiencing fear. It can really help for you to understand that your emotion is fear, to stay with it, breathe into it and let it be. The feelings of fear are there, because your system wants to protect you. It will be important that you take action in those areas in which you can, but at the same time learn to accept that there will be aspects over which you have little control. Staying with your fear and observing it, as an emotion, rather than fighting it will in the long run be a more helpful approach.

# SADNESS

Everyone experiences sadness from time to time and it is also a very common emotion associated with HIV infection. Sadness is common if you are rejected, excluded or disliked, or when you are with others who are in pain. Sadness is also experienced if you lose something that is important to you. Some people living with HIV who were diagnosed in the mid 1980s have experienced multiple losses of partners and friends. Sadness may be easier to bear if the loss is temporary, for example, if a close friend is away for a while, but much, much harder if it is permanent, for example the death of a loved one.

Sadness very often arises during transitions or changes in our lives. This is because transitions nearly always involve losses, as well as, gains. Being diagnosed HIV positive can be thought of as a transition, involving losses and gains through which you need to navigate. For example, it is not uncommon for people to say that while their diagnosis represented a loss, they made changes to their lives that have been gains, such as considering their own needs as equal to others or learning to be more honest or take better care of their needs.

# ANGER

Anger is an emotion that usually occurs in response to a boundary violation. You may have encountered situations in which you were insulted, violated disrespected, physically or emotionally hurt, threatened or you did not get something, which was very important to you or you got something that you didn't actually want. In all these situations anger might be felt. Anger can be directed at other people or at yourself, in the form of internalized anger, or both at the same time.

Anger is another common emotion associated with HIV. When you first learn of your HIV status it is not uncommon for people to say that they feel angry with themselves, other people or their situation. It is often the case that anger arises in situations where you also experience helplessness Sometimes, the anger might even cover up deeper underlying feelings of fear or sadness. For example, if a partner rejects you, your anger about this might cover up your underlying feelings of fear about being alone and the sadness over the loss. It is important that you understand and recognize your anger, but not act on it in a way that could be harmful to yourself or others.

## SHAME

Shame is yet another common emotion associated with HIV infection, as there is often an assumption that people will blame you for contracting the virus. It has been given a lot of attention in recent years. It is known that people who experience high levels of shame have poorer mental health, partly as they tend to be more isolated. Chapter 4 on disclosure and stigma looks at this important emotion in more detail.

Shame feelings are often generated in social situations and are associated with automatic thoughts that others see you as inferior, bad, inadequate and flawed, which feels as if others are looking down on you with a condemning or contemptuous view. This may lead you to become self-critical and self-attacking if you believe them.

The emotions and bodily feelings generated by shame are various, but include anxiety, anger and disgust in the Self and self-contempt. Shame is often seen as the opposite to pride. Shame is related to weakness and loss, but has also been linked to loss of dignity and (dis)honour. Shame often binds (or fuses with) other emotions such as anxiety, anger or disgust, giving different textures to how it is experienced.

Shame is often associated with specific defensive behaviours, such as a strong urge to 'not be seen', avoid exposure, to hide, and/or run

PART
A

PART
B

PART
C

away. Eye gaze is commonly averted and you may feel inhibited from responding spontaneously to another person.

SELF-MONITORING: A CHANCE TO CHECK-IN WITH YOURSELF • *emotions associated with HIV* (1) *Firstly, can you think of times during which you have experienced emotions in relation to HIV? What were those emotions? Did you experience any of these strongly, frequently – which ones? (2) Secondly, check-in with yourself to reflect on: How you have managed emotions that may have felt unhelpful or stressful to experience in the past? What behaviour did you use to manage such emotions? Notice what made it better or worse for you? It could be very helpful to write these down in your diary, notebook or on a sheet of paper, so that you can later decide on what might help you to manage your emotions well.*

PART
A

PART
B

PART
C

# CONCLUSION

There are many reasons why, as human beings, it is useful to experience emotions and they are both essential to our survival and unavoidable. In relation to HIV a wide range of associated emotions can occur due to the impact it can have on your life and relationships. It is important that you acknowledge that some degree of emotional reaction is completely normal and part of your adjustment process. The more you learn to understand, allow and accept your emotional reactions, rather than resisting them, the easier it will be for you as they are a valuable source of information to you.

For some people, emotions can feel too intense and unmanageable in relation to HIV. The next chapter will focus on some of these more problematic emotions and how these express themselves. The emotional strategies listed in the next chapter are developed to help you in dealing with them.

PART
A

PART
B

PART
C

# 8

When Emotions are Difficult

# INTRODUCTION

The previous chapter outlined the nature of emotions and those that may be triggered due to being diagnosed as HIV positive. Emotions are clearly a normal aspect of being human, however, you may find that sometimes they feel unmanageable or unbearable. Many people say that when they were diagnosed with HIV, their sense of loss and fear felt unmanageable for a period of time. You have probably found that like most people feelings become much harder to cope with, when they are very strong, it seems as if you have no control over them, and they stop you from doing what you need to do, like concentrate. What you feel, and how strongly you feel it, depends on many things, and in this chapter we will attempt to help you develop your understanding of your own feelings and the way they work.

Most people living with HIV infection say that being diagnosed was one of the hardest things they ever had to cope with in their lives. It is understandable therefore that you may need a lot of support during this time in your life. Remember, emotions signal to you that something has happened in your life, which has had an effect on you. The experience may have affected you in a positive or a negative way and emotions help you notice and understand the effect that any one experience has had on you. While there are always individual differences in how people respond to the same life event, some life events are more distressing than others. Studies have suggested that the most stressful events in ranking order are (1) death of a partner, (2) separating from a partner, (3) a jail term, (4) death of a close family member, (5) personal injury or illness, and (6) being made redundant.

At this time a good social support system can be extremely helpful to you. Social support refers to having relationships, in which you can confide and talk about your emotions in a supportive way and perhaps gain some practical assistance at times. Frequently this type of support can be provided by people like friends, family members and partners, but it could be anyone who you feel can help you during this time. The important thing is that you feel supported by the relationship and this can help you greatly to cope with difficult emotions. The most important aspect when thinking about social support is the quality of the relationships you engage in rather than the quantity of them. It will be far more helpful to you to have a few very close relationships, in which you feel supported, rather than many casual relationships, where trust has not been sufficiently established. If the latter describes you, you may like to consider, which of these more casual relationships might have the potential to develop into closer, more trusting relationships, in order to bring more support into your life during this time.

The following chapter highlights some of the times when HIV can become quite difficult to deal with. The areas of emotional invalidation, secondary emotions, recreational drugs, self harm and suicide will be focussed on. In this book, we draw especially, but not exclusively, on the work of an American Psychiatrist, Marsha Linehan, who we would like to acknowledge as having worked over several decades with people on understanding and overcoming difficult feelings as part of her development of a therapy called Dialectic Behaviour Therapy (DBT).

# EMOTIONAL INVALIDATION

HIV is a condition that can make you emotionally very sensitive to judgements from others around you. These may be actual judgements from others or judgements, which you perceive to be there. Both can put you in touch with feelings of shame and stigma, which are painful to carry. The way you relate to other people is therefore very important. People will vary in their level of ease in relation to trusting their emotions and expressing them as a result of their social learning and experiences. It is important to remember that every person is entitled to experience and express their own emotions. However, this also includes you and it is important that you do not allow other people to judge you or put you down for having 'your own feelings'. Frequently expression of these can be hard enough in our society, where emotions to this day are often considered uncomfortable and avoided, but recognising when people invalidate your own emotions, can help you overcome this.

Emotionally invalidating experiences are those in which:

- Your feelings are ignored, neglected or punished
- The expression of emotions is met with erratic
  or inappropriate responses by others
- Your understanding of your feelings,
  behaviour, or situation is dismissed
- You are treated as if you are to blame for your feelings and
  should be able to control them and not show them
- Problems in life including emotional distress are attributed to
  negative personal characteristics attributable to yourself, by others
- Solutions to problems in life, including emotional
  distress are oversimplified by others

It is worth recognizing that most of us will have been exposed to a certain amount of invalidation by others, either when we were children, teenagers, or also during adulthood. We would like to invite you to reflect for a minute and think about how emotions were dealt with in your family when you were growing up. Were feelings expressed freely within your family or were they rarely talked about? Were expressions of distress met with a warm and caring response from your parents or were they met with a critical reaction like *"boys don't cry?"* or a reaction that made you feel stupid and ashamed? We have observed that the way parents talked to their children when they were upset is often reflected in the attitudes people hold towards their own feelings. We all engage in self-talk, which is thinking to ourselves in our inner mind about our experiences. If you find that your self-talk can be very self-critical towards your feelings, then it probably resembles the voice of your parents or others important past authority figures. This is because children and young people tend to internalise the voices of others so that in later life it feels that they have become your own. Recognising the sources of critical self-talk can be the first step towards adopting a more compassionate and nurturing stance towards your feelings.

When we are children and our emotions are invalidated, we tend to feel bad for having these emotions. Usually, we start to seek the blame within ourselves and try to block how we feel or at least not to show these emotions to others, because we learn that they are undesirable. Therefore, we often learn quite early in our life that our emotions are not valid or to be trusted and should not be expressed. Unfortunately, when we are young, we seldom recognize that there was nothing wrong with our emotion or our emotional expression. We do not understand that when our emotions are invalidated, this has usually more to do with the person who invalidates our emotions, rather than with the emotion itself or the emotional expression of this. Mostly, invalidation happens when another person can't bear to hear our emotions, possibly because they feel helpless, overwhelmed or unable to cope with emotions. Frequently this is because they themselves have not learnt to express their emotions. This way the invalidation of emotions is perpetuated and passed from generation to generation, so that it influences the whole of our society. With time, you may yourself have learnt to invalidate your own emotions. Therefore when people are judgmental towards you, you may feel bad and you may be quite easily prepared to invalidate your own emotions, which then makes you feel bad and makes your feelings much harder to experience. The key is therefore to be aware of how others treat you in relation to how you are feeling. It could be helpful for you to understand that their invalidation of your emotions is more likely to be related to their own difficulties with emotions. It is also important for you to become aware of how you treat yourself in response to other people's difficulties in coping with emotions.

PART
A

PART
B

PART
C

EXERCISE *What do you think about the following exchange? Alan: "I've been feeling pretty depressed for the last few months. Things with my partner are not going well and my $CD_4$ count continues to drop. The doctor says I will have to think about starting combination therapy." Paul: "All you need to do is to think more positively." Alan: "What do you mean?" Paul: "Well, rather than focusing on the negatives, just focus on the positives!".*

How would you be feeling if you were Alan? Do you think Alan would feel supported and validated by Paul's responses? The answer, as you've probably already thought, is "no". Let's examine why. The underlying message coming from Paul is that the reason Alan is feeling depressed is not because of the obvious threats to his relationship and his health, but because he is not thinking positively enough. Paul's suggestion that the solution to Alan's problems is to think positive is a huge oversimplification. If the solution were that simple, no doubt Alan would have implemented it already! Paul's responses are an example of emotional invalidation. He may not be being intentionally malicious, but unable in this example, to deal with Alan's distress. This is likely to be related to Paul's own difficulties in dealing with Alan's situation. Therefore it is important that Alan doesn't feel bad about being depressed and invalidates his emotional response, but that he seeks support from someone other than Paul, who would be better able to help him express and validate his emotions.

Other examples of emotional invalidation in relation to HIV include:

- You tell your friend/partner that you're feeling overwhelmed, because of the issues that being HIV+ create. They look at you and reply that at least you're not working at present, so what's so stressful?
- You explain to your partner that you are still feeling side-effects from the HIV drugs. They respond by saying that you are lucky to be on treatment.

It is important, whenever you encounter experiencies of emotional invalidation, to recognize these and stop yourself from moving into feelings of shame or blame. Remind yourself that it is understandable that you are experiencing difficult emotions in relation to various factors in your situation and that you are perfectly entitled to experience these. Allow yourself to seek support from people, possibly also considering the work with a Clinical Psychologist or an Accredited Psychotherapist, who can understand, accept and explore your feelings.

# SECONDARY EMOTIONS

In the previous section, both primary emotions and secondary emotions were outlined. Primary emotions are those that are felt as a direct consequence of a certain problem or situation. A primary emotion is, for example, the depression that Alan experienced in the previous exercise in response to his current condition of having HIV. Secondary emotions are usually a response to primary emotions and are emotions in their own right. They can be a product of us responding to others invalidating us, as was explained in the previous section. For example, when you judge yourself negatively in response to other people's invalidations of your primary emotions, the feelings that arise for you subsequently in relation to your self-judgements are secondary emotions. These often occur automatically and you may not be aware of their detrimental effect on you, which will be further explored in this section.

PART
A

PART
B

PART
C

The self-invalidating judgements that produce these secondary emotions can ultimately lead to emotional escalation. Allow yourself to look at the example in Figure (19) on the next page.

In this example, someone is rejected by another person, because of their HIV status. One of the emotions that this inevitably triggers might be anger. Another emotion may be sadness, but for the sake of this example, anger especially will be focussed on. Obviously being rejected, because of HIV status is difficult enough in itself. However, if additionally, you internally judge yourself about feeling angry your emotional distress escalates even further. Often these judgements contain the word "should", as shown above.

"Should" judgments are usually accompanied by blaming statements such as: "I'm pathetic or weak". Often they will reflect the way others around you when you were young did not accept your feelings or

PART
A

PART
B

PART
C

```
            ┌─────────────────────────────────┐
            │        TRIGGERING EVENT          │
            │   Rejection because of HIV status │
            └─────────────────────────────────┘
                          ⬇

            ┌─────────────────────────────────┐
            │        PRIMARY EMOTION           │
            │             Anger                │
            └─────────────────────────────────┘
                          ⬇

            ┌─────────────────────────────────┐
            │      EMOTIONAL ESCALATION        │
            │      (SECONDARY EMOTIONS)        │
            │    Anger +++, shame, anxiety     │
            └─────────────────────────────────┘
                          ⬆

            ┌─────────────────────────────────┐
            │        JUDGEMENTS CAUSE          │
            │       SECONDARY EMOTIONS         │
            │   "I should pull myself together" │
            │   = feeling angry about feeling angry │
            │   "I'm pathetic for feeling like this" │
            │   = feeling ashamed about feeling angry │
            │   "I can't cope, this will overwhelm me" │
            │   = feeling anxious about feeling angry │
            └─────────────────────────────────┘
```

Fig. 19 Example of secondary emotions

attacked you for having them. Other types of judgement can be fears about not being able to cope with emotions, as outlined above. You are more likely to make these judgements if you have had experiences of being undermined in the past. These judgements usually also contain predictions about the consequences of your emotions, such as being overwhelmed, or losing control. It is important therefore to monitor your secondary emotions, as they can increase your level of stress. Engaging in self-judgement and the secondary emotions it produces, leads to emotional escalation. Figure (19) highlights how this can happen. It is useful therefore to learn how to defuse from your judgements and not become entangled in them, by noticing that your mind is producing judgements and carrying on with what you need to do.

The focus, so far, has been on emotions that might be called "negative", such as, sadness, anger and fear, and the type of judgements associated with them that lead to emotional escalation. However, it is also the case that emotions known as "positive", such as, happiness and excitement can be associated with judgements that can be problematic. For example, if you do not experience positive emotions very often, sometimes you may want to hold on to them when you feel them. Happiness may be longed for and when experienced may lead to judgments that can lead to secondary emotions, which can overtake the primary emotion as is shown in Figure (20) on the next page.

In summary, this section indicates the importance for you to become aware of your secondary emotions in response to the primary emotions you may experience. Generally, the more you can allow yourself to experience and acknowledge your primary emotions, without moving into secondary emotional responses, the more helpful it will be to you. Emotions can be painful and difficult to handle, however, by moving into secondary emotions, you are likely to escalate your emotional distress rather than soothe it. If you observe that you might be moving into secondary emotional responses rather often and find that you can't move yourself out of them, you may like to consider professional help for learning to cope with your emotions more constructively.

PART A

PART B

PART C

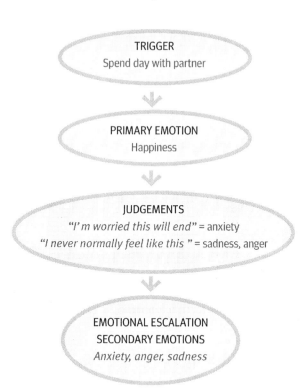

Fig. 20 Another example of secondary emotions

# OTHER SELF-LIMITING STRATEGIES PEOPLE USE TO TRY TO MANAGE FEELINGS

## USING RECREATIONAL DRUGS TO COPE WITH HIV-RELATED EMOTIONS

Recreational drugs, such as, cannabis, ecstasy and cocaine are widely available. The same is true for alcohol. Many people feel that alcohol and recreational drug use does not result in any serious problems. However, recreational drugs and alcohol have very strong effects on how people feel. In the short term, they can sometimes make people feel happier very quickly. Many people have therefore at some points in their lives used drugs and alcohol to deal with emotions. If they knew of other ways to manage their emotions then it would be unlikely that they would have come to rely on recreational drugs or alcohol. If you find yourself relying on these to manage emotions, you are more likely to use alcohol and recreational drugs in a way that could be harmful to you, especially in the longer term.

Figure (21) illustrates how getting drunk results in the temporary alleviation of problem emotions. This coping method, however, results

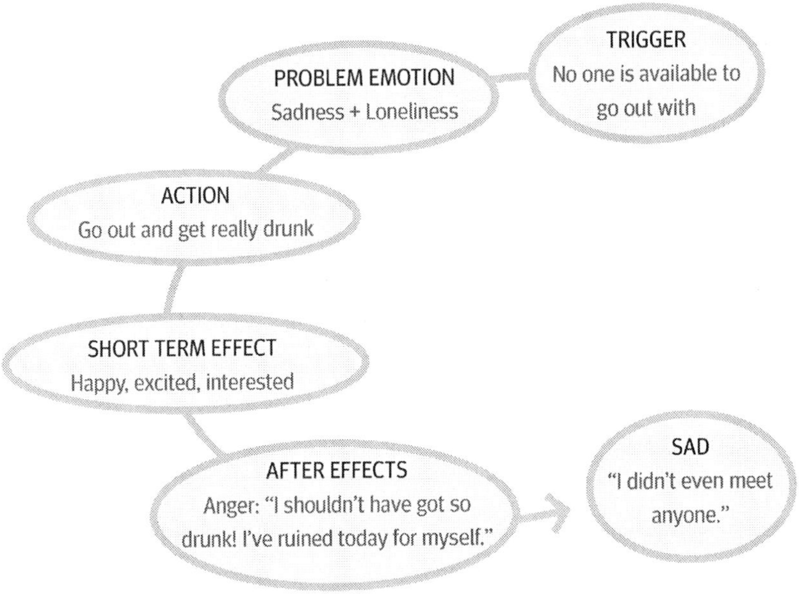

PART
A

PART
B

PART
C

**TRIGGER**
No one is available to go out with

**PROBLEM EMOTION**
Sadness + Loneliness

**ACTION**
Go out and get really drunk

**SHORT TERM EFFECT**
Happy, excited, interested

**AFTER EFFECTS**
Anger: "I shouldn't have got so drunk! I've ruined today for myself."

**SAD**
"I didn't even meet anyone."

Fig. 21 Using alcohol to cope with emotions

in more problem emotions the following day, which subsequently increases the likelihood of getting drunk in order to cope even more. It can also cause you secondary problems; because of the disinhibition you may be experiencing at the time when you are intoxicated.

## SELF-HARM

We all experience changes in our mood, but for some people they find it very difficult to keep control over their behaviour and experience, because their mood feels very difficult and different at times. If you are someone who finds that how you feel about yourself is unstable and that you can switch from one state of mind where for example, you feel intense anger, to another where for example, you feel emotional blankness, unreal or muddled, then this section might be particularly useful to you.

If this is the case you may be attempting to cope with these very strong emotions and sudden changes in mood by doing things that other people may find difficult to understand. One of these might be self-harm. Self-harm is usually thought of as a deliberate attempt to inflict injury or pain to your body by, for example, cutting, burning or hitting.

The main reason why people self-harm is to cope with intolerable and unbearable emotional pain. Self-harm can seem very effective, temporarily, in reducing distress, as it can help to distract from the original emotional pain. However, if you do self-harm it is usually, because you do not know other less harmful ways to manage your emotional pain. Therefore your episodes of self-harm are your means of coping with your emotional pain. However, although this may afford you temporary relief, the personal costs of this strategy can be very high. This way of coping does not take away or alleviate your emotional pain. It only temporarily displaces it with more immediate bodily pain or injury, which requires your attention. It is also a strategy that people use who feel very disconnected, emotionally empty or dissociated from themselves. Self-harm, in this instance, may be your only way to experience any feeling at all. However, if this is the case for you, the costs of this strategy can be high. It is also possible that you learnt this strategy of self-harm in order to cope with other earlier, very painful experiences in your life. There are many more healthy alternative strategies of coping with your emotional pain or with your feelings of inner emptiness or dissociation, which you could discover and use instead. Even if you have used this strategy for a long time, now may be the time in your life to learn different and healthier strategies of coping. You may, however, need some professional help with this.

If you or someone you know is affected by self-harm there are many sources of professional help and advice, which you could access for support. You may benefit from psychotherapy. For example, Dialectical Behaviour Therapy (DBT) or Schema Therapy (ST), both forms of Cognitive Behavioural Therapy for more complex problems, could help you learn more healthy coping strategies. If you have experienced traumatic experiences early in your life, specialist therapy for complex trauma, such as Positive Growth Therapy (PGT) or Sensory Motor Therapy (SMT) may also be helpful for you. There are some resources for this listed in the Appendix of this book.

## SUICIDE

Suicide is the conscious, deliberate and purposeful taking of your life. It is associated with intense emotional difficulties and inner turmoil. Self-harm is different from suicide in that the usual function is to control emotional pain, rather than to end your life, although this may be an unintended consequence.

PART
A

PART
B

PART
C

Suicidal thoughts and behaviour are much more common than most people think. For example, about 10% of the UK population will have attempted suicide. It is also known that suicidal thoughts, attempts, and fatalities are more common among people living with HIV infection than in the general population.

A common trigger for suicide is often intolerable psychological pain. People who are suicidal will usually be feeling extremely hopeless and helpless about their situation and can see no way out. The common intention of suicide is often to seek a solution, where no other solutions are perceived to exist. While ultimately, it is difficult, if not impossible, to prevent a person who is really intent on committing suicide, often people can be helped out of these dark periods in their lives. Appropriate and often professional support during these times can create new hope for a suicidal person and recognition that other solutions exist, which at the time were not available to the person seeking to commit suicidal action. Suicidal actions also communicate anger and distress to those around and are extremely distressing and frightening not only for the person intending to commit suicide, but also for those close to them. With appropriate support and intervention from health professionals many suicide attempts can be prevented. If this applies to you or a person you know, it would be very helpful to seek the support of an appropriate professional resource, such as, a Clinical Psychologist or an Accredited Psychotherapist.

### SELF-MONITORING: A CHANCE TO CHECK-IN WITH YOURSELF * *difficult emotions* ( I ) *Firstly, can you think of times when you experienced difficult emotions in relation to being HIV positive? What were these emotions like and how did you experience them? Were these difficult emotions the result of*

*someone emotionally invalidating you or of your own secondary emotions? (2) Secondly, how did you manage your difficult emotions? Did you use unhelpful strategies or helpful strategies? It could be very helpful to write these down in your diary, notebook or on a sheet of paper, so that you can later decide on what might help you to tackle your difficult emotions.*

# STRATEGIES TO REDUCE
# THE STRENGTH OF YOUR EMOTIONS

The current context of your life can influence how you respond emotionally. Certain factors may make you more vulnerable to experiencing your emotions as more overwhelming and making you feel less able to cope with them. Therefore, understanding and counteracting some of these factors could be very helpful in reducing your vulnerability to difficult emotions, when they arise in response to specific triggers. These factors include:

PART
A

PART
B

PART
C

- The amount of sleep you are getting. Sleep deprivation increases emotional vulnerability.
- Alcohol and recreational drugs. These are mood altering and can make it harder to regulate your emotions.
- Amount of exercise you are giving yourself. Exercise has been proven to improve mood and can therefore reduce emotional vulnerability.
- Diet. Maintaining a balanced and healthy diet can help with your emotions.
- Balance. Attempting to keep some kind of balance over the various commitments in your life can help maintain emotional

health. Working all the hours that exist by contrast leaves little time just for you and increases your emotional vulnerability.

- Stress. If you are stressed and having to deal with many life events this may result in emotional fatigue.

Below is an outline of a range of specific strategies that can be applied to help you manage difficult emotions.

## (1) ACCEPTANCE

You cannot control and resolve every aspect of every situation. Having ups and downs in your life is part of the human condition. However, you have choices about how you cope with the things, which you cannot change or control. For example, you cannot control the weather, but you can choose what to wear. You cannot control whether the train arrives on time, but you can decide what to do while waiting for it. If your train is late you may think: "*it should be on time*" and feel frustrated. If you continue to think this over and over again, while having no control over the situation, you will become more and more frustrated.

Refusing to accept the reality of a situation can increase your level of stress and distress. For example, when someone loses their partner they are often in great emotional pain. Initially, it is often difficult for a person to accept that they have no control over such an event. People are often overwhelmed by the great sense of loss that they experience and their emotional response to it. However, if they continue not to accept what has happened as time goes by, their pain can turn into suffering, that is, pain plus the non-acceptance of pain and a resulting struggle that leads nowhere, as there really is no way of changing the situation.

You may find it very difficult to accept the reality of your HIV infection when you are first diagnosed. Often people say: "This cannot

PART A

PART B

PART C

be happening to me!", or: "This should not be happening to me!", or: "Why did I not protect myself?". This is an understandable response for some time following your initial diagnosis and indicates that you are still in shock and can't quite comprehend what has happened. However, if you continue to say these kinds of things to yourself over a longer period of time, it makes it much harder for you to let go of the distressing emotions associated with your HIV diagnosis.

Accepting something does not mean you have to approve of it. You do not have to like something in order to accept it. Acceptance is partly about acknowledging the degree of control or lack of control that you have over something. It is partly about acknowledging that you cannot turn the clock back and that you have to deal with the reality of the here and now. It also means accepting your emotional responses to the situation and carrying on regardless with living the life you want. Figure (22) summarizes the effects of acceptance versus non-acceptance.

PART
A

PART
B

PART
C

|  | ACCEPTANCE | NON-ACCEPTANCE |
|---|---|---|
| SITUATION | *Acknowledge* | *Deny* |
| CONTROL/ NO CONTROL | *Do something Don't fight* | *Do nothing Hit head against a brick wall* |
| EMOTION | *Self-validate* | *Self-invalidate* |

Fig. 22 Acceptance vs. non-acceptance

# (2) SELF VALIDATION

Being judgemental towards your emotions can make matters worse. It is important to notice when you are being judgemental towards your own emotions. Writing an emotion diary is one way of getting some distance from your emotions and crucially, identifying judgements towards your own emotions. Look at the "emotion diary" in Figure (23), below, with some examples where we help identify the primary and secondary emotions with the associated thoughts and think about ways of challenging them with more positive and realistic thoughts.

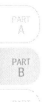

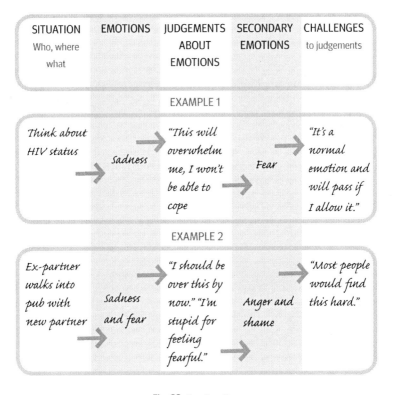

| SITUATION<br>Who, where<br>what | EMOTIONS | JUDGEMENTS<br>ABOUT<br>EMOTIONS | SECONDARY<br>EMOTIONS | CHALLENGES<br>to judgements |
|---|---|---|---|---|
| **EXAMPLE 1** | | | | |
| Think about HIV status | Sadness | "This will overwhelm me, I won't be able to cope | Fear | "It's a normal emotion and will pass if I allow it." |
| **EXAMPLE 2** | | | | |
| Ex-partner walks into pub with new partner | Sadness and fear | "I should be over this by now." "I'm stupid for feeling fearful." | Anger and shame | "Most people would find this hard." |

Fig. 23 Emotion diary

Try completing an emotion diary yourself using a recent time when you had a difficult emotional experience. You may initially find it hard to separate the experience into the above components for a number of reasons. Both the primary and secondary emotions can occur at the same time. The primary emotions can be very quickly replaced by the secondary emotions. Also, for some people the secondary emotions can be much stronger than the primary. Watch out for "judging your judging", i.e., becoming concerned about how well or badly you are doing and being critical of what you come up with.

Once you are able to identify the judgements you are making about your primary emotions, the next thing is for you to understand the kind of theme they reflect. Identifying the theme will enable you to think of alternative responses, which you might then like to use instead.

## (3) IF YOUR THOUGHTS CONTAIN "SHOULDS"

If you are telling yourself that you *"should"* not to be feeling the way you are you will most likely be invalidating yourself. If you are finding it difficult not to become entangled in your judgements try to validate your emotions instead. Most of the time your primary emotions will be telling you something about yourself, or some aspect of your situation. Certain primary emotions tend to be associated with certain kinds of events. Think about your emotions and the situation and they will often make sense. Asking yourself the following questions in a kind and uncritical manner may help you to do this:

(A) **"Are these emotions surprising given the circumstances?"** HIV is a potentially life threatening infection. Is it surprising therefore that people sometimes experience fear associated with infection? If someone lost a partner who meant the world to him or her, is it surprising that they sometimes experience sadness years later?

**(B) How would other people feel if they were in a similar situation?** Think about the kind of things that tend to upset other people or that you have observed to upset them. For example, if you know other HIV positive people, chances are you would have talked to them about the time when you learnt of your diagnosis or other common experiences and found your emotions were similar to theirs at the time.

**(C) What would I say to a friend if they were feeling this?** People are notorious for having one (usually harsh) rule for themselves and one (usually tolerant) rule for others experiencing emotional pain. If someone close to you were feeling the way you are feeling, what would you say to them to comfort them? If you are not finding it easy to think about what you would say to a friend, think about what you would say to a child if they were feeling the way you were. Check that the rules that you are applying to yourself are also kind and fair to yourself.

## (4) IF THEY CONTAIN "I CAN'T COPE"

Sometimes emotions can feel as if they will overwhelm you. People may think that an emotion that causes discomfort will go on and on. You may have in the past coped in a way that was harmful. Past experience though is not necessarily a good guide to model future experience. If a certain emotion tends to lead to a certain pattern of behaviour this might suggest thinking or doing something different in relation to it. The following may be useful in deciding whether your fears about being overwhelmed or not coping could be reassessed.

**(A) How long will an emotion last?** People often overestimate the length of a difficult emotion – because emotions can be so painful they can feel as if they will last forever. While it takes longer for some people's emotions to return to normal than it takes others, all emotions are time-limited. The fact they can quickly re-occur can make it feel as if they have never stopped.

**(B) What can I do to manage this emotion?** It is easy to forget all the things you can do to influence the emotion, as emotions affect the way you think (see below). Writing short lists of things that you can do to manage emotions, which you already know work and are easily available, can be useful. For example, there are many ways to divert your attention away from your emotions. You may find things like hitting a pillow, listening to your favourite music through headphones, or running on the spot, can help reduce the intensity of an emotion. It can be useful to do some research, while not in the grips of an emotion and see what kinds of things suit you best. For example, if you're a keen jogger then running might be more easy to remember and more likely to work.

**(C) Was there anything you learnt the last time?** Think really hard about the last time an emotion was difficult. Was there anything that seemed to make the slightest bit of difference to you? If so can you do more of this next time when you have to confront a difficult emotion?

# (5) ACTING IN THE OPPOSITE MANNER TO THE EMOTION

Emotions may trigger urges for you to take action. You may get caught up with the feeling, as well as, the urge to take action. Figure (24) lists some common emotions, their "action urges", and the opposite action you could chose to take instead. Acting opposite to the emotion requires you to be aware of the emotion and its action urge, and choosing and implementing a different course of action.

There are some points to bear in mind that will help you decide whether it is helpful to use opposite action to manage emotions:

- **Firstly, only use this when it makes sense.** For example, if a stranger in a bar makes you afraid, it may be more appropriate not to confront them and leave rather than stay.
- **Secondly, use this when your emotion is unfounded.** For example, you may be angry with a friend for turning down a date, because they could not find a childminder. In this case, your response of anger would be unreasonable and it would be helpful for you to understand why you are responding in this way. Rather than attacking your friend, in this situation it will be helpful to be kind to your friend and yourself.
- **Thirdly, do not use the opposite action if it would reinforce the emotion and/or lead to difficult secondary emotions.** For example, being passive when angry and in danger of attack may make you feel weak and more vulnerable to attack.

PART A
PART B
PART C

| EMOTION | ACTION URGE | OPPOSITE ACTION |
|---|---|---|
| Fear / anxiety | *Avoid or flee* | *Expose to fear until it subsides* |
| Sadness | *Inactivity or withdrawal* | *Energise, do things that give mastery and pleasure* |
| Shame / anger | *Hide and disappear* | *Initiate, make eye-contact* |
| Anger | *Attack* | *Be kind, de-escalate* |

Fig. 24 Acting the opposite to the emotion

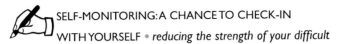

**SELF-MONITORING: A CHANCE TO CHECK-IN WITH YOURSELF** • *reducing the strength of your difficult emotions (1) Firstly, when you have experienced difficult emotions, have you ever attempted to reduce their strength? If so how? If not why not? (2) Secondly, check-in with yourself to reflect on: which strategies suggested in this chapter could you use to manage and reduce the strength of your difficult emotions? It could be very helpful to write these down in your diary, notebook or on a sheet of paper, so that you can later decide on what might help you to tackle some of these.*

# CONCLUSION

The greater your level of emotional arousal the harder it will be for you to tolerate your feelings. Everyone at some point in life will have responded to an emotion in a way that, on reflection, may not have been the most effective or helpful. Part of being human is accepting that we are not perfect and sometimes what we do in the heat of the moment has unintended consequences later that are not always welcome afterwards. If this has happened to you, then it is important to take responsibility for your actions and the consequences that may have arisen without being judgemental toward yourself. It is helpful to develop a more compassionate and accepting stance toward yourself and your circumstances. This applies also to your emotions and your ability to acknowledge and carry them. As a general rule the stronger the emotion you experience, the more dramatic the action needed to bear it. That is why finding healthy and constructive ways of dealing with your emotional flames is so very important.

PART
A

PART
B

PART
C

# Mindfulness and HIV

# INTRODUCTION

The previous chapters explored the nature of emotions, relating to them and difficulties associated with them. This chapter covers the skill of mindfulness. This skill can help with difficult emotions in its own right.

Mindfulness is a novel approach to emotional acceptance. Its origin can be traced back to as early as the first millennium B.C., to Buddha, the founder of Buddhism. It is now being widely used by Psychologists and used to help many people. Acceptance of having HIV and the difficult emotions and situations that it can raise is often a problem for people who are HIV positive, and mindfulness provides a way of being with yourself that will help you deal with what life brings you.

PART
A

PART
B

PART
C

# MINDFULNESS – WHAT IS IT?

Mindfulness is best explained by an example. If you drive, you will have experienced driving to a certain place and realizing you have gone the wrong way, only becoming aware of having done so until some time later. Non-drivers will have experienced the same when walking. This common phenomenon highlights several things. It shows that our minds have a habit of taking us to places where we do not always want to go. It also illustrates that we may not be aware that our mind has done this until later. It shows that we do not have to be aware of what our mind is doing for it to influence us. Not being aware of what your mind is doing is the opposite of mindfulness.

It is obviously really useful to have an aware and clear mind and in many situations this is helpful. However, in order to optimize the use of our mind it is helpful to learn ways in which we can train it, a bit like a muscle, to perform in certain ways. As the example, above, illustrates if we don't attend to what our mind does, it can take us away from what is actually happening at the present moment in time. At best this leads to feeling disconnected from our surroundings and at worst this could even expose us to harm, as you may not have paid attention to a situation, which in actual fact presented an advantage or a disadvantage to you.

MINDFULNESS has been described as "paying attention (to your mind) in a particular way: on purpose, in the present moment, and non- judgementally".

Mindfulness enables you to be aware of the nature and contents of your mind and how it is affecting you. Being mindful enables you to stand back and gain distance from your thinking so that you can attend to the moment, observe and describe it. It puts you back in touch with your observing Self that is not caught up in the contents of language, definitions and judgements, and is a source of wisdom and calm.

It also enables you to look at your thinking from an observer position rather than become caught up in it. It is increasingly recognised that our mind can take us to places that generate difficult emotions and body sensations without us being aware of how it has done so. Most people will have experienced an apparent "inexplicable" change in their mood. This is an example of your mind being able to influence your mood without you being aware of the cause. This is because we can only process a certain amount of information in consciousness at any one time. Other information is processed out of our awareness or unconsciousness. But this does not mean the information is not important or the processing will not have an effect on you. Those of you with experience of meditation will notice some similarities between the practise of meditation and mindfulness.

# MINDFULNESS HAS SEVERAL APPLICATIONS

(1) It can help you increase your awareness of difficult emotions and the processes underlying them. In other words, it can help you know what is "going on" inside your mind. Once these processes are identified, action can be taken. For example, it can help you identify the judgements you make towards your emotions that lead to making them more difficult. It is not a distraction technique, using it in this way is simply another avoidance measure that leads back to the pain you may be trying to avoid. If negative feelings come up, just notice them and keep on doing what you were doing.

(2) Mindfulness can also be used to disengage from distressing thoughts and emotions. We can easily fall into distressing negative patterns of thinking, particularly when depressed or anxious. These patterns have the characteristics of being incredibly repetitive and self-critical, using almost all of your attention, and leaving you feeling that you are at the mercy of your thoughts and feelings. This form of thinking is called *rumination* and serves no helpful function, although most sufferers may think it does and find it very difficult to disengage from it.

Ruminative thinking is usually the result of some mismatch between how you think things ought to be or would like them to be and how things actually are. For example, HIV positive people may say to themselves: "I shouldn't have got HIV!", which can trigger ruminative patterns of thinking that can lead to fierce self-recrimination.

PART A

PART B

PART C

You may attempt to cope with rumination by trying to think your way out of it. For example, if someone has the thought: *"I am a failure because of HIV"*, they may respond with *"I am a good person, HIV+ or not"*. This exchange can go on and on. It's a bit like the equivalent of the pantomime exchange of: *"Oh no he isn't – oh yes he is!"*. Similarly you might try and tell yourself: *"...not to think about it!"* that only makes you think about it more. What is often more helpful than these styles of coping is a way of switching your mind into a different mode or activity.

In mindfulness you observe and describe mental activity without avoiding it. This is done non-judgementally, calmly, in a focussed way and without doing other things at the same time.

SELF-MONITORING: A CHANCE TO CHECK-IN WITH YOURSELF • *what is mindfulness? (1) Have you ever heard of 'mindfulness' or realised that it can be a helpful psychological way of 'being'? Does it make sense to you that you can still be in yourself but also observe yourself at the same time? (2) How does it feel to know that you can use mindfulness as a way to manage emotions? Think of situations when inner calmness or stillness has already been helpful to you. It could be very helpful to write your responses down in your diary, notebook or on a sheet of paper, so that you can later use these as you learn and apply mindfulness.*

# OBSERVING WHAT YOUR MIND IS DOING

If you are going to be able to describe the process and content of your thinking, it is important to be able to get some distance from it. This can be difficult particularly during periods of strong emotions when you may experience the belief that all that matters is the contents of your mind and how physically uncomfortable or tense you may be feeling as a result. Practising observing what your mind is doing without getting stuck on the content of your thoughts is one way of gaining objectivity from it and staying in the present.

> 👉 EXERCISE | *Maintaining attentional control. Sit or lie somewhere comfortable. Make sure it is quiet. Breathe slowly in and out through your nose. Do this until you have established a rhythm. Shut your eyes. The task is to focus all your attention on your breathing – the flow of air going in and out. Do this for a couple of minutes. If your attention wanders, gently bring it back to your breath. Stop and write down what you noticed.*

PART
A

PART
B

PART
C

## EXPLORATION

Most people when they first try this notice that their mind wanders constantly onto other things such as other sounds in the room, a conversation earlier that day, what's happening later, thoughts about how well they are doing the exercise and so on. Even if someone is in the room reminding you to focus on your breathing, most people find their mind quickly wanders. This exercise shows (1) how your mind has "a mind of its own", and (2) how you do not always notice where your mind has gone! This usually takes you away from what you are actually doing in that moment, which may well be free from difficulty and possibly keeps you dwelling in a difficult place in the past or future.

## POSSIBLE APPLICATION

With practice it should become easier to notice when the focus of your attention has shifted to something else and therefore to bring it back to what you want to focus on. You can develop your own versions of this exercise like focusing on the lyrics in a song.

This could include focusing your attention on different parts of your body that are usually out of awareness like your toe, knee, little finger, etc. Focus on how these parts of your body are feeling with an open, curious mind, rather than judging these feelings in any way. Or you could count your out-breaths up to the count of seven and return to one, and then keep repeating this over and over. The key is to focus on something and then notice when your attention has shifted and bring it back. Being able to sustain and shift the focus of your attention at will in an accepting and observational way will help you be able to cope better when troubled by distressing thoughts or emotions. It will help you feel less at the mercy of them and increase your confidence in handling difficult emotions.

In addition, if you are having difficulty sleeping as a result of your thoughts racing, as they do in the ruminative mode of mind, you may find this exercise a useful way of shifting your attention away from the contents of your mind and towards your breathing and thus making it easier for you to fall asleep.

EXERCISE 2 *Observing the contents of your mind. This exercise is more concerned with watching your thoughts so you can then describe them. This requires staying in the present and not letting your mind take you elsewhere, which was the purpose of Exercise 1. Make sure you are sitting or lying in a quiet and comfortable place. Shut your eyes. Watch out for your thoughts and emotions as they come and go, just like the waves rolling in from the sea onto a beach. Do this for a few minutes. Write down what you noticed.*

## EXPLORATION

People vary tremendously in what they observe when they do this exercise. You may observe lots of thoughts coming and going, or very few. You may observe emotions, such as happiness, sadness, or anger. You may also observe how they affect your body and breathing. Occasionally, you may find your thoughts are racing so much, that you have not been able to "catch" any thoughts. This may have the effect of tensing your body up and your breathing becoming faster and shallower.

If you are having difficulty observing your thoughts, there are other ways you can try and achieve this. For example, you can try and imagine projecting your thoughts onto a screen as if they were film titles, or you could write your thoughts down. The only point of this exercise is to observe what comes up without any judgement or expectations. If nothing comes up then all you need to do is notice that.

## POSSIBLE APPLICATIONS

With practice, the exercise should make it easier to observe your thoughts and emotions, and the effect they have on your mind and body. This has many benefits. It will make it easier for you to be aware of what you are thinking and feeling. It will also make it easier for you to identify things that cause problems, such as emotional judgements. During periods when your emotions are running high, getting some distance from them can help cool the situation down a little.

# DESCRIBING WHAT YOUR MIND IS DOING

Noticing what your mind is doing is an important step towards being mindful. But you also need some way of describing what you observe.

The principle is to describe what you observe non-judgementally. Thinking *"I'm a bad person"* is being judgemental towards the Self. Describing the same thing mindfully and non-judgementally would be to say, *"A thought that "I'm a bad person" just entered into my mind"*. Describing emotions with phrases like *"I'm sad"* or *"I'm angry"* implies you are your emotion. It is not possible to become your emotion. When emotions are very strong they can often feel like facts. Emotions are things people experience. It is important to try to describe them mindfully. For example, *"A feeling of anger/sadness has just welled up inside me"*, or if experiencing shame *"I feel like I want to hide from everyone."*

# DOING ONE THING
## AT A TIME, INCLUDING MINDFULNESS

Life can be full of competing demands on your time and it can be difficult for you to fit everything in. Often people do more than one thing at a time, such as eat while watching the television, write on the computer while talking on the telephone, and so on. If you do more than one thing at a time, you cannot be giving it your full attention. The amount of attention you give to something influences your experience of it. Try these little exercises.

- Choose a piece of food. It doesn't matter what. It could be a raisin, an apple, a sweet, etc. Make sure there is nobody and nothing to distract you. Shut your eyes, place the food in your mouth and concentrate by focusing all your attention on eating. Pay attention to the smell, the taste, and the texture of your experience. Eat and chew very slowly. Try to capture the whole experience. You will never have thought that eating a raisin (or whatever you chose to eat) could be such a (relatively) profound experience!

- Try reading a story in a mindful way and notice whenever you find your mind wandering away. Just observe where it goes and if it is to a thought, name it as such in a non-judgemental way, and bring yourself back to the text. If something is going on in the room that takes your focus, name what you are doing, for example "looking", and bring your attention back to the book.

If you do not give something your full attention, you may miss something important. Attending to emotions in a focussed way can alter the nature of the experience for the better, and give you a greater opportunity to notice the content and processes of your thinking and emotions, and then have greater choices in how you react to situations.

PART
A

PART
B

PART
C

# MINDFULNESS IS NOT CONCENTRATION

Concentration is when you focus your mind on one thing, such as, when you are removing a splinter from your finger. Concentration requires will power to force the mind to focus on something. Without concentration, there cannot be mindfulness; however, there is a distinct difference between them. Concentration focuses attention; mindfulness determines upon what the attention will be focused and detects when attention strays. As Figure (25) shows, there are three aspects to mindfulness that make it distinct, namely, Meta-awareness, being Undistracted and Non-judgemental.

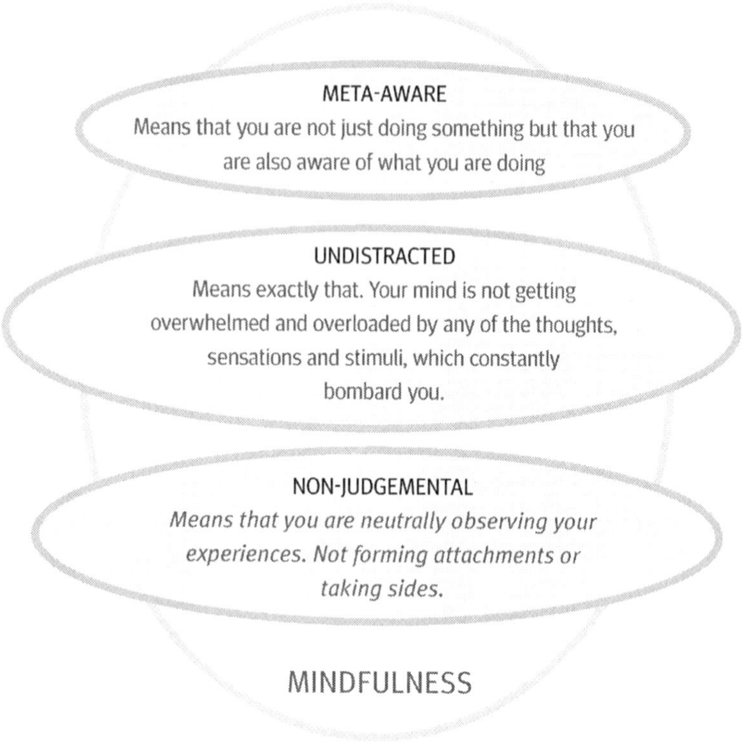

**META-AWARE**
Means that you are not just doing something but that you are also aware of what you are doing

**UNDISTRACTED**
Means exactly that. Your mind is not getting overwhelmed and overloaded by any of the thoughts, sensations and stimuli, which constantly bombard you.

**NON-JUDGEMENTAL**
*Means that you are neutrally observing your experiences. Not forming attachments or taking sides.*

MINDFULNESS

Fig. 25 Three aspects of mindfulness

# USING MINDFULNESS WITH DIFFICULT EMOTIONS

As we have stated, there are many difficult emotions associated with HIV. Examples of these include: receiving news from your doctor that your viral load has increased; hearing people speak negatively and inappropriately about HIV; or, feeling overwhelmed when you think about disclosing your HIV status. At these times you may feel disturbed, angry, anxious, hurt and so on. Instead of judging your emotions, avoiding them or reacting to them, (i.e. doing what you would habitually do), you may like to try the following, using the mindfulness techniques in this chapter:

Mentally observe your reactions
Notice what it feels like in your body
Notice and stay with your bodily feelings
Notice and stay with the emotions and what you are feeling
Don't suppress or fight any of what comes up for you
Accept your bodily feelings and what they do
Accept your emotions
Be present with your emotions and feel them
Wait until your emotions pass

A useful way to remember the above, especially when you may be overwhelmed with emotion, is by using the 'wave metaphor'. To illustrate this: a surfer surfing on the sea does not fight the waves, as the waves are unavoidable. Instead, the surfer rides the waves and goes along with them, thus not avoiding their uncontrollability. In a similar fashion, you can become submerged and overwhelmed by your bodily reactions and your emotions. So if you become overwhelmed by your experiences – surf them, don't fight them.

PART
A

PART
B

PART
C

# TAKING MINDFULNESS FURTHER

This section was intended to give readers a flavour of mindfulness, its practice and uses. If it has caught your interest there are plenty of ways of taking it further. A good starting point is to practice yourself and there are lots of resources out there, such as books and tapes to help you do this. If you decide you would like to experience mindfulness directly, the most effective way of doing this is to receive training by an experienced teacher. Information about courses and a whole lot more can be found at www.dharma.org. Mindfulness is closely connected to Buddhism and many practitioners of mindfulness will also be practising Buddhists. You do not have to become a Buddhist though to practice mindfulness or Buddhism, as it is open to anyone.

 SELF-MONITORING: A CHANCE TO CHECK-IN WITH YOURSELF • *being mindful (1) Firstly, did you attempt the mindfulness exercises suggested in this chapter? How did it feel, what was it like? What did you observe? (2) Secondly, check-in with yourself to reflect on: When could you start to use these strategies during your normal day? When you are travelling on the bus, walking down the street, eating your dinner, thinking about yourself, thinking about being HIV positive? It could be very helpful to write these down in your diary, notebook or on a sheet of paper, so that you can later expand on some of these further.*

# CONCLUSION

It is inevitable that there will be times when you experience high levels of bodily and emotional distress and you will not know what to do or where to turn. There may also be times when the way you have coped with an emotion leaves you with some difficult feelings afterwards.

Mindfulness is one of an array of useful techniques that can help you deal with approaching difficult emotions or bodily reactions in a healthy, positive manner. It is useful to practice the skill of mindfulness with easy things like eating a raisin or managing your breathing. Only when you have mastered these will you be able to apply mindfulness to more complex things like managing emotions or complex feelings. Mindfulness essentially can become a totally new way of being with yourself in the present, which enables you to experience life far more fully and aware.

PART
A

PART
B

PART
C

# 10

Strategies for Anxiety and Depression

# INTRODUCTION

This chapter focuses on anxiety and depression, as they are the most common psychological problems in the general population. We have already briefly looked at them in Chapter 2. They are, however, especially common for people with HIV and because of this need extra attention as they can become quite overwhelming and distressing. We will help you, firstly, to recognise whether you are feeling these states and explore why. We will then, secondly, suggest helpful strategies that are based on a symptom-management approach to dealing with anxiety and depression that focuses mainly on your thoughts and behaviour.

PART
A

PART
B

PART
C

# WHAT ARE THE SYMPTOMS
# OF ANXIETY AND DEPRESSION?

For you to be able to recognise whether you are anxious or depressed you will need to be able to identify the basic symptoms that you will experience in your body when you may be in these states. Everyone feels depressed and anxious to some degree, at different times in their lives. You may therefore have experienced the symptoms to varying degrees already. The following table in Figure (26) lists the main symptoms that can be grouped into four main areas, namely:

# HOW TO MANAGE ANXIETY AND DEPRESSION

You can see that there are many warning signs of anxiety and depression, falling into the four categories, we highlighted. We suggest that the

| | ANXIETY | DEPRESSION |
|---|---|---|
| **PSYCHOLOGICAL SYMPTOMS** The way your mind responds to experience | Scanning the environment for possible sources of danger Fearful thoughts, reduced reasoning ability Loss of confidence Feeling inadequate Difficulty concentrating and focusing | Less ability to think or concentrate Loss of sex drive Loss of confidence or self-esteem Recurrent thoughts of death or suicide Feelings of hopelessness Increased self criticism and feelings of guilt |
| **BEHAVIOURAL SYMPTOMS** What you may do or not do | Panic driven behaviour Increased vigilance and watchfulness Avoidance of situations Restlessness | Decreased motivation to do things Avoidance Slowing down Social withdrawal |
| **PHYSIOLOGICAL SYMPTOMS** How your body feels | Increased heart rate Feelings of faintness and/or dizziness Increased startle reaction Shallow fast breathing Decrease in appetite | Disturbed sleep, for example, early morning waking 2 hours or more before the usual time or difficulty rousing at all Body feels numb/shut down Feeling more easily tired Increase or decrease in appetite |
| **EMOTIONAL SYMPTOMS** How you feel | Worry Feelings of uneasiness and foreboding that something bad will happen Fear Feelings of overwhelm Loss of confidence | Loss of interest or pleasure in activities that are normally pleasurable Lack of emotional reactions to events or activities that normally produce an emotional response Emotional disconnection from people who in the past felt close Feelings of hopelessness and despair |

Fig. 26 Anxiety and depression symptoms

key to managing these if you experience them is to think of a particular symptom that bothers you, and which you wish to resolve, and then pick out the strategy that is the most appropriate for you from the ones we will now describe.

For example, if you are experiencing uncomfortable thoughts in relation to HIV you could attempt to challenge them and find alternatives, or problem-solve the concerns, which you are experiencing. Alternatively, if you are feeling physically tense you may benefit from relaxation. Below, is a list of possible symptom-based techniques aimed at symptom-reduction that you could choose from when you experience distress?

SELF-MONITORING: A CHANCE TO CHECK-IN WITH YOURSELF • *feeling anxious and/or depressed (1) Firstly, as different symptoms can present in different people, which of the above symptoms of either anxiety or depression have you ever experienced in the past or do you experience currently? Are there any particular types of symptoms that you experience often or feel more concerned about? (2) Secondly, what have you attempted to do already to help lessen the symptoms that you have had or may be currently experiencing? Has what you have done helped? It could be very helpful to write these down in your diary, notebook or on a sheet of paper, so that you can later evaluate further what might help you to tackle some of these*

# (1) RELAXATION

This is useful for calming physical symptoms, such as an increased heart rate and light-headedness by helping you let go of the muscle tension that occurs as a result of anxious thoughts. It also helps you breathe more effectively and helps to calm the flow of distressing thoughts, which keep coming into your mind by distracting you from these and focussing your attention on the present.

You may like to try the following in addition to the techniques described in Chapter 2:

(1) Lie down and try to let go of any tension you are feeling in your body. Then focus on your breathing and feel the air as it comes in and out of your nostrils. Notice the temperature of your breath as you breathe in and the temperature as you breathe out. As you do this if there are any thoughts interfering, don't fight them, just acknowledge them and then let them go. Allow yourself also to let go of any body tension you may have. Do so for at least ten minutes.

(2) Lie down and focus on your breathing until you have reached a steady calm rhythm. Then imagine your body being a block of ice as a result of the tension, which you are holding. With each out-breath imagine the ice melting, as you focus on each part of your body, in turn. Start with your head, move to your neck and shoulders, arms, back, stomach, buttocks, thighs, calves and then your feet, leaving your muscles feeling physically relaxed and invigorated. Enjoy the feeling of softness in your body, as you are feeling increasingly relaxed.

## (2) DISTRACTION

This is a useful strategy for when distressing thoughts keep coming into your mind, as sometimes switching your attention to something more pleasant and immediate can be helpful. Why not try these:

* Focus on an object that takes your attention, such as, a flower or a painting and describe it to yourself in as much detail as possible.
* Focus on a pleasant memory, for example, of a calm, peaceful

natural setting you may have visited, like a beach or a meadow.

* Ring a friend.

* Read a book or try and write your own story.

* Play some music, sing a song.

* Engage in an activity, such as going shopping, watching an uplifting film, doing a crossword or sudoku, playing a game, such as solitaire, going swimming or for a walk in a nice place.

## (3) GRADED EXPOSURE

If you are finding yourself avoiding events, situations or experiences, due to fear or hopelessness, then you may like to plan gradually facing those situations in a safe way, especially if you realise you are missing out on something you may value, such as, social contact. For example, if you are not going out, because you are worried about people asking you about yourself and having to hide your HIV status.

Here is what you might try and do to tackle your avoidance:

* Think about a possible situation that applies to you and work out what conditions could make it easier for you to deal with this. You might feel that the avoided situation would be easier to deal with if it involved greater or lesser time with people, more or less people, different times of the day, people you know better than less well and so forth. Consider the particular situation you have avoided and write down as many factors, as occur to you that would make it easier for you to attempt it.

* Start with the situation that would be easiest for you to handle. For example, start with meeting those people you could manage the easiest, such as, arranging to have coffee with a friend who has HIV in the daytime. Allow yourself to face this situation and explore

PART
A

PART
B

PART
C

if the fears, which you have had about socializing are the same as the reality that you encounter in this situation. For example, the person may not ask you awkward questions about your status or appearance as you had feared, or if they did, you actually find yourself being able to deal with these better than you had feared, or the other person came across as non-judging and accepting, which was quite different to what you had feared. Experiences, which are different in reality from what you had feared, will then enable you to become more adventurous. They can enable you to try increasingly difficult social situations and increase your feelings of confidence about you being able to face them. It can also be very helpful for you to rehearse in your imagination these scenes, but if you do this, it is important to visualise positive outcomes rather than rehearsing the negative ones. Allow yourself to think about how you would cope in a positive way even with a situation that was difficult for you.

- Repeat facing your fears in a safe way with increasingly difficult situations until it does not create anxiety for you anymore. By doing this in a gradual way, starting with the easier and only advancing to more difficult situations, when you feel you can comfortably tackle a harder situation, you can overcome your avoidance. Be sure to praise yourself or acknowledge your achievements as you progress through your avoided situations.

## (4) SCHEDULING ACTIVITIES

If you are depressed this may be partly because your life feels full of things you don't enjoy, you feel out of control of, or you are doing too little to give your life value. A worsening cycle of doing less and less can set in making you feel more depressed. A way out of this is to realise you are doing this and plan activities that counteract this pattern of events:

* Keep a diary of what you do for a week and work out whether you are doing enough activities that you enjoy and feel in control of. Of course there may be some things you need to do that you would rather not, or things you can't do because of restrictions, such as, that they are too expensive. On the whole we are looking for some balance in your life where you are at least spending some time doing enough of those activities that you value.

* If you find out that you are not doing this, plan things to do that are meaningful and fulfilling for you on a daily basis. You could get a member of your family or a friend to help you think of activities that are enjoyable and join in with you. This could be anything from exercising, working, supporting a worthy cause in some way, shopping, cooking, pursuing a craft, to walking in nature, looking after an animal and much more. These activities could be more action-oriented or more contemplative, depending on what you feel would be most helpful to you. Sometimes, finding activities, which enable you to connect to the person within, such as joining a Tai Chi, Yoga or meditation group can be very helpful.

* Initially it may take some effort to make yourself do things, but if you can persevere with this it will break the cycle of depression by giving you back hope and enjoyment in your life.

## Behaviour and Breaking Cycles

Both anxiety and depression are influenced by and can influence your behaviour. At a simple level, it is what you do or what you don't do that counts. Figures (27) and (28) demonstrate this point.

The depression diagram (figure 27) illustrates that when you are feeling depressed, your level of interest goes down. This, of course, then influences your level of activity, which tends to decrease. If you do

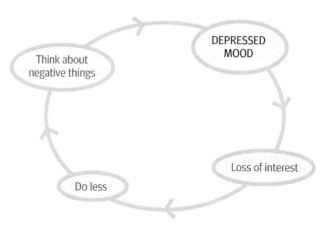

Fig. 27 A vicious cycle model of depression

PART
A

PART
B

PART
C

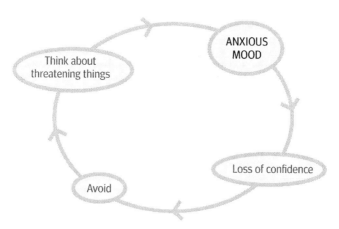

Fig. 28 A vicious cycle model of anxiety

less, then you are likely to feel that either life is not very stimulating and has little of value to offer or you devalue yourself for not being more active. Either way, it is likely that the intensity of your depression increases. If you do less, you also have more time to ruminate about negative things, which, in turn, is likely to exacerbate your depression.

A strategy you could use to get out of this negative, downward spiral would therefore be to do more. Similarly with anxiety, the same pattern can emerge, namely that a person can feel anxious, which affects their level of confidence. Then, they avoid situations, which confirms their feelings of incompetence and increases the time to think anxiously and this then reinforces the level of anxiety.

These two diagrams illustrate how people can get trapped into unhelpful cycles of behaving that maintain the depression and anxiety. Challenging and breaking these cycles can make all the difference.

## (5) PROBLEM-SOLVING

Problem solving is useful for dealing with things that worry you, which can have solutions. It gives you a method for working things out by breaking a problem into smaller and more manageable parts with suggestions on how to deal with them. As this is covered extensively in Chapter 11, we will only briefly mention it here. Problem solving can help you to:

- Think of the problem and list the steps needed to reach a goal that will help address the problem.
- Reward yourself for each step or goal that you have achieved.

## (6) ENLIST SUPPORT

Depression and anxiety can result from you feeing isolated and unsupported by others. Creating a social network can help you change this (also see Chapter 3):

- Find someone you trust and talk to them about your concerns.
- Maintain social contacts, such as friendships or family.
- Attend groups to meet people who may be in a similar situation to you.

## (7) CHALLENGING DISTRESSING THOUGHTS

If you are distressed or anxious, your thinking may be rather negative and unhelpful and contributing to the emotional problem. Most people think in this way from time to time, but when you are extremely depressed or anxious your thinking may actually be keeping you in that state. We will look at some of these styles of thinking in more detail (HIV cognitive distortions), but challenging some of your more distressing thoughts in a kind and positive way can help to weaken the strength of belief you may have in them and reduce your distress:

- First identify the distressing thoughts you are having.
- Question these thoughts and look for evidence for and against them.
- Think about whether someone who you trust would agree with them.
- Think about the effect that these thoughts are having on you and whether there may be a more helpful thing to say to yourself.
- Think about what action you could take to disprove them or to get you out of the situation of dwelling on them.
- You might also want to ask yourself when these thoughts started and whether there is any underlying reason for why you are tormenting yourself with such thoughts. For example, the thoughts may have started when you did or didn't do something or if you feel guilty about something. As you become aware of the underlying reasons for your feelings, acknowledge your discovery.

# THINKING AND THINKING STYLES

*Men are not worried about things, but by their ideas about them. When we meet with difficulties, become anxious or troubled, let us not blame others, but rather ourselves, that is, our ideas about things.* Epictetus (1st Century AD)

This quote sums up the final part of this chapter, namely, that the way we perceive things, situations, events can influence the way we feel. However, the way we feel then influences our thoughts and beliefs. Figure (29) shows this relationship between events, thoughts and mood.

Despite overwhelming amounts of information we have in our environments to make sense of the world, the following exercise shows just how easy it is to make an assumption and act upon it.

EXERCISE *Read the short story, below, carefully and when you've finished try and answer the question, without looking at the text again. "An empty bus leaves the depot for the day's run. On the first stop, it picks up 10 people...the next stop it picks up 20 people...then it lets off 15 people at the next stop... after this 30 people are picked up...then it lets off 20 people...at the next stop it picks up 15."*

The question to the exercise is: "How many stops did the bus make?" Did you feel able to answer the question straight away? If not, why not?

* You may have made an assumption thinking that the question would be about the number of passengers.
* That assumption then would have affected the way in which you

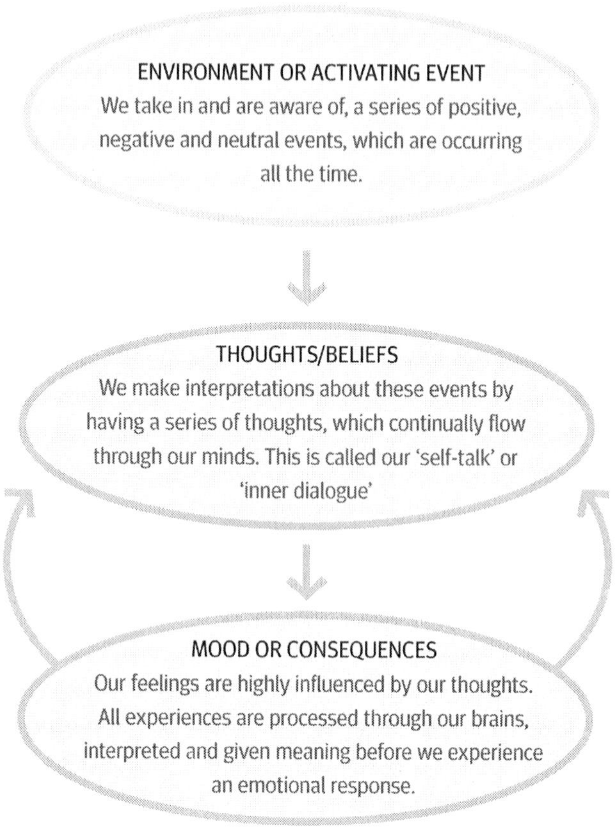

PART
A

PART
B

PART
C

## ENVIRONMENT OR ACTIVATING EVENT

We take in and are aware of, a series of positive, negative and neutral events, which are occurring all the time.

## THOUGHTS/BELIEFS

We make interpretations about these events by having a series of thoughts, which continually flow through our minds. This is called our 'self-talk' or 'inner dialogue'

## MOOD OR CONSEQUENCES

Our feelings are highly influenced by our thoughts. All experiences are processed through our brains, interpreted and given meaning before we experience an emotional response.

Fig. 29 The relationship between events, thoughts and mood

behaved, i.e. which aspect of the story you attended to. You listened to the information in a way that was consistent with your original belief about what the question would entail, such as how many people are on the bus rather than how many times did the bus stop.

● That assumption was wrong in this case. This exercise shows just how easy it is for all of us to act upon a belief that may not be accurate and from there drawing the wrong assumptions. Do you find you have many assumptions relating to having HIV? For example, how people will see you and react to you?

# HIV-RELATED COGNITIVE DISTORTIONS

If you are depressed or anxious, it can alter your beliefs and the way you see the world, yourself and other people. As Figure (29), above, showed, mood can arise as a consequence of your thoughts, but it also can affect your thoughts.

Thinking styles in anxious and depressed people can become distorted and may not reflect the reality of a situation. If you are anxious you are likely to think more fearful thoughts than if you were not anxious. If you are depressed you may think more hopeless thoughts about having HIV and your future than if you were not depressed. These thought distortions are types of mood-related thinking styles that can really get you down. In order to be able to cope with them you need to be able to recognise and challenge them or accept them for what they are (merely thoughts) and not believe in them.

To illustrate how you could experience thought distortions with HIV, the following are examples of common faulty or unhelpful beliefs in relation to HIV that people can have. As you can imagine they can influence how you react to and cope with situations rather a lot. Therefore recognising them can help you to prevent the problems from getting worse. Most of the beliefs have a grain of truth in them, but are distorted in some way to make them partly or wholly inaccurate, as

PART
A

PART
B

PART
C

they are clouded by emotions. The key to coping with these thoughts is to challenge or accept them for what they are, as shown in each of the comment sections, below.

## (1) BLACK AND WHITE THINKING

You view a situation in strictly black and white terms (a complete success or a total failure) without seeing the shades of grey. This is also called polarized thinking.

EXAMPLE: A friend who you recently disclosed your HIV status to has not contacted you for a longer period than usual. You think this can only mean that they have changed in their perception of you and are uncomfortable about you being HIV positive.

COMMENT: There are lots of reasons why they may not have phoned, yet. You have not checked it out with them. You may be assuming that everyone will reject you, because you have HIV, including your friend. You might like to take action and call your friend to check out how they are and whether there is any problem in your relationship with them as a result of your recent disclosure.

## (2) OVERGENERALIZATION

You allow an isolated event to indicate to you that this event will always represent similar situations everywhere, related or unrelated. You therefore draw a sweeping negative conclusion that goes way beyond the present situation.

EXAMPLE: When spending the evening with your family you hear some of them being critical about a man with HIV on the news. You conclude that all people hate people who are HIV positive and that you'll always be rejected.

COMMENT: It may have been the detail of the story that made them sound judgemental. Have you checked this out? Some people's uninformed attitudes do not represent all people's views! Sometimes it takes time for people not to be afraid of HIV. Despite the fact that ignorance exists, there are many good accepting people. What about the times you have heard others commenting about HIV positively and with respect?

## (3) FORTUNE TELLING

You predict the future (or recent past) negatively, usually catastrophizing with little or no evidence to base this on.

EXAMPLE: Despite being in good health and on HIV antiretroviral drugs, you still conclude that you will always have health problems and will die from HIV very soon.

COMMENT: In reality how can anyone know about what tomorrow will bring for them. It is definitely known that people are not dying of HIV related illnesses in the same numbers as they used to. Your fears may be clouding your judgement of reality and stop you from living the quality of life you could enjoy in the here-and-now.

## (4) MIND READING

This is the magical gift of being able to know what someone else is thinking without the aid of verbal communication! You therefore believe that you do know what others are thinking and how they view a situation without verbally communicating with them.

EXAMPLE: In a social gathering, you just feel that the people you are with 'know' that you are HIV positive. This makes you feel increasingly uncomfortable and you hide away in a corner all evening.

COMMENT: People cannot read minds and know the medical

PART
A

PART
B

PART
C

histories of the people they are with, without reading through their medical file. You are jumping to conclusions about what others are thinking as this is clearly a sensitive issue for you.

## (5) MAGNIFICATION and MINIMISATION

You make a situation out to being much worse than it is or play down the severity of a situation. You see a circumstance in greater or lesser light than is appropriate.

EXAMPLE: You see having HIV as meaning that you are worthless as a person, and that others can never be accepting of you.

COMMENT: No one with HIV is worthless. HIV is only a part of you and your life – what about all the other things that make you, you? What about everything you have achieved in your life up to this point? What about the talents and skills that you have and that make you unique as a person?

## (6) LABELLING

You use a mistaken judgement of yourself to define yourself. You put a fixed, overgeneralized label onto yourself or others based on little evidence.

EXAMPLE: You see yourself as unlovable and unable to have a sexual relationship just because you are HIV positive.

COMMENT: There are many opportunities for you to have meaningful relationships when HIV positive. You are equating one aspect of yourself with a global negative statement about yourself.

## (7) EMOTIONAL REASONING

This is where you think something is so true, just because you believe it to be true.

EXAMPLE: You believe that your life will be over as you have HIV.

COMMENT: Your life is different now, but not necessarily completely and negatively changed. What is the evidence that your life is over? Remember that society is more accepting about HIV and people are living for longer!

*SELF-MONITORING: A CHANCE TO CHECK-IN WITH YOURSELF ● recognising and changing your thoughts (1) Firstly, cognitive distortions are common for most people. Did you recognise any of the listed HIV-related cognitive distortions? What sorts of HIV-related cognitive distortions do you experience most frequently? (2) Secondly, check-in with yourself to reflect on how you may attempt to deal with these thoughts? Do you attempt to challenge your negative thoughts? What successes have you had? It could be very helpful to write these down in your diary, notebook or on a sheet of paper, so that you can later decide on what might help you to tackle this further.*

PART A

PART B

PART C

# WHAT ARE HELPFUL AND UNHELPFUL BELIEFS?

What you believe can help or hinder your way of coping with having HIV. The following Figure (30) shows how to recognise what a helpful belief is, as opposed to an unhelpful one, which may be based on emotional thinking, for example, as a result of you feeling depressed or anxious. The seven HIV thought distortions listed, above, are all examples of unhelpful beliefs. The seven accompanying comments are examples of helpful beliefs. If you learn to recognise these patterns in

239

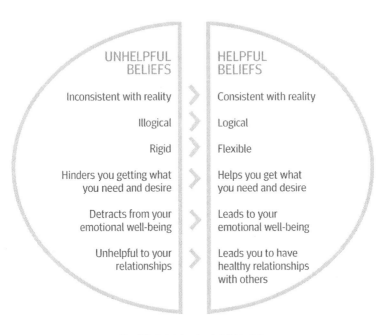

| UNHELPFUL BELIEFS | | HELPFUL BELIEFS |
|---|---|---|
| Inconsistent with reality | > | Consistent with reality |
| Illogical | > | Logical |
| Rigid | > | Flexible |
| Hinders you getting what you need and desire | > | Helps you get what you need and desire |
| Detracts from your emotional well-being | > | Leads to your emotional well-being |
| Unhelpful to your relationships | > | Leads you to have healthy relationships with others |

Fig. 30  Helpful and unhelpful beliefs

yourself it will help prevent you believing in something inappropriate and unhelpful to you.

# CONCLUSION

This chapter has focused on the typical symptoms of anxiety and depression. It has outlined strategies that can help you, with particular reference to what you may do and think in relation to having HIV. The strategies are symptom-based and problem-focussed. They require some practice and you need to tailor them to the specific needs in your particular situation. When you have not thought about things in this way, before, it may take you some time to apply some of these changes. If more positive, reality-based thinking doesn't come easily to you at first, don't give up, but be patient with yourself. Persevere in trying out different strategies and try and identify those which are most helpful to you. It could also be helpful for you to write down when a strategy has worked for you, so that you can draw on it again in the future. Alternatively, you may want to seek the help of a Cognitive Behavioural Psychotherapist or a Clinical Psychologist to help you start with this process, if you find that you are not advancing further with this on your own.

PART
A

PART
B

PART
C

# 11

# Problem Solving and HIV

# INTRODUCTION

Problem solving is a strategy that you can easily learn and use in order to help reduce the distress associated with problems you experience in your life. As highlighted in previous chapters the need to accept, validate and understand your emotions is important in helping you cope with HIV. Problem solving can be most useful when there are practical things that can be done about your situation. It doesn't really matter what the problem is, as the approach is normally the same.

Problem solving can be used time and time again. Why is problem solving a helpful strategy? Well, it is logical, systematic and a reasonably easily learned approach to finding a way out of a situation. It also has the advantage of being based on common sense principles. So it will help anyone. People who have been found to be good problem solvers have been found to cope well with life's ups and downs. This chapter will focus on this technique.

PART
A

PART
B

PART
C

# WHAT IS PROBLEM SOLVING?

Problem solving:

- Identifies problems as causes of distress.
- It helps you look at the resources you possess for approaching your problems. It teaches you a systematic method of overcoming current problems.
- It enhances your sense of control over problems.
- It equips you in a preventative manner, with a method for tackling future problems.

SELF-MONITORING: A CHANCE TO CHECK-IN
WITH YOURSELF • *conversations about solutions ( I )*
*Have you ever thought about how important it is to start having*
*'conversations about solutions?' You can have them internally with*
*yourself or with another person. (2) Try to talk about yourself in*
*a 'problem-free way', focusing on what you have achieved, what*
*resources you have and what you are capable of. Try to have*
*conversations about yourself regarding past successes in solving or*
*coping with problems, current partial solutions and ways to amplify*
*these successful actions in the future. It could be very helpful to write*
*these down in your diary, notebook or on a sheet of paper, so that*
*you can later come back to these.*

# THE SIX STEPS TO PROBLEM SOLVING

If you follow the six instructions, below, you will find that problem solving really makes things seem less overwhelming and more manageable.

## STEP 1

*What is the problem?* Identify and define clearly what the problem is. What do you worry about? What gets you down? What would you rather be doing without? What do you need help with? Examples of HIV-related problem areas are listed in Figure (31).

It can be seen that there are many areas of your life where problems can occur. Try and think of what these are for you. You may have several problems so you can look at them one at a time.

## POSSIBLE PROBLEM AREAS

- Your relatonship with your partner or finding a partner
- Your relationship with your family
- Your ability to negotiate your health care system
- Your disclosure of HIV to significant others
- Your emloyment/studies/hobbies
- Your finances
- Your housing

- You legal position
- Your social isolation and relationships with friends
- Your use of alcohol and drugs
- Your psychological health
- Your physical health
- Your sexual adjustment
- Beareavement and impending loss

**Fig. 31** A vicious cycle model of depression

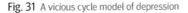

PART
A

PART
B

PART
C

# STEP 2

*List all possible solutions – even bad ones!* Think of as many ways as you can that could address the problem. At this point it doesn't matter if some are not such good solutions; the point is that you think of as many solutions as you can. The more you try to think of solutions the more you will find!

# STEP 3

*List the advantages and disadvantages of each solution.* There will always be good or bad aspects to addressing problems with particular solutions. The point here is to think reflectively about what will be good and bad for you. Try and bring this to paper, as it will help you to see the advantages and the disadvantages of each solution clearer.

## STEP 4

*Choose the best solution or combination of solutions.* Decide on which option or options are realistic and unrealistic.

## STEP 5

*Plan how to carry it out.* Choose the option that is both most rewarding and feasible. Prepare and plan ways of undertaking the chosen option. Plan how to carry it out and when you will carry it out. Set yourself a realistic time frame, within which you want to achieve your chosen option. Write this down for yourself.

## STEP 6

*Take action and praise all efforts.* Now undertake what you have planned. Whatever you do, be proud of what you are doing! Praise yourself after you have taken action, even if further action is required to achieve the desired outcome. Be kind and patient with yourself.

# PROBLEM SOLVING AND HIV

Problem solving is useful, because it is helpful in negotiating the many issues that can evolve in HIV and that can at times be overwhelming. Due to the range of your constantly evolving needs, service changes, demands of treatments and so on, you can often feel overwhelmed with the issues that you need to negotiate. Problem solving just helps you to divide tasks and breaks them down, so that they can feel more manageable and achievable to you.

The following list illustrates the issues in HIV, which you may encounter, that may be helped by your use of problem solving. You may experience many or only a few of those issues listed, below, at different times:

- Disclosing HIV to family or friends
- Negotiating whether to work or study
- Coping with health problems
- Enjoying a safe sex life
- Managing to take HIV medicines without trouble
- Coping with mood problems
- Communicating effectively with medical staff

Bob *was diagnosed HIV positive a month ago. The only people he has talked to about HIV are the staff at the hospital. He has started to feel very lonely and wants someone he trusts in his life to know his diagnosis so that he can get informal support. He realizes that he needs to disclose his HIV positive status to someone but needs somewhere to start working this out.*

The completed problem solving exercise sheet on the next page shows how Bob has, at this point in his life, and at this stage in his awareness of HIV, used problem solving to help him disclose to someone.

SELF-MONITORING: A CHANCE TO CHECK-IN WITH YOURSELF • *practice problem solving (1) Have you got a problem in your life at the moment? Do you want to reduce the existence of the problem and the effect it has on your life? Chose something relatively easily manageable, when you are trying this for the first time! (2) Use the empty problem-solving sheet, below, and following on from Bob's example above, identify a particular problem that you are experiencing in your life at the moment. Work out the steps you could take to resolve that problem. It could be very helpful to write these down in your diary, notebook or on a sheet of paper, so that you can later evaluate how the process of problem solving went for you.*

## PROBLEM SOLVING
### HIV Disclosure – Bob's Example

**Step 1. What is the problem?**

*(1) I have not told anyone about my HIV positive diagnosis*

*(2) I feel that I should at least tell some people who are close to me. Who should I tell, how should I tell? Should I tell?*

*(3) I am scared to tell anyone, because of how they may react to me!*

**Step 2. List all possible solutions – even bad ones**

*(1) I can just tell my best friend*

*(2) I can tell all my friends*

*(3) I can just tell my mother*

*(4) I can tell all of my family*

*(5) I can tell my neighbour*

*(6) I can tell my children*

**Step 3. List advantages and disadvantages of each solution**

*(1) My best friend – I've told him other problems, surely he will understand me*

PART
A

PART
B

PART
C

(2) All my friends – what is the point of telling them, it is not the worlds' business!

(3) My mother – well I am very close to her, I want her to know everything about me.

(4) All of my family – many of them I don't see very often and I actually don't like Uncle John, so I am reluctant to tell them.

(5) My neighbour – well I get on with her, but is it really her business?

(6) My children – they are too young to understand. Maybe in the future.

## Step 4. Choose the best solution or combination of solutions

(1) My best friend – I've told him other serious problems, surely he will understand me

(2) My mother – well I am very close to her, I want her to know all about me

## Step 5. Plan how to carry it out

My best friend: I will remind myself that I know that there is nothing wrong with me, whatever people say about me being HIV positive. I will hold on to this knowledge whatever the outcome of the disclosure. I will tell my best friend when we are out together next week. We often like to go to that quiet bar to talk. I have helped him at times so he should help me now. I actually feel safe about telling him, because he talked about someone who was HIV positive and didn't say anything bad about them.

*My mother: I will tell my mother the next time we are alone, when I visit her at her house. My mother has always told me that she will stand by me whatever life brings. I have to tell her and when I do I will try to remain calm and answer her questions. I will be prepared for her to be a bit shocked at first.*

Step 6. Take action and praise all efforts

# CONCLUSION

You can now see how problem solving works and that it is quite easy to do. There are so many new aspects to your life when diagnosed with the HIV that it can just feel too overwhelming. Problem solving therefore can help you to make your life much more manageable. It can help you to feel more in control of your HIV related issues.

Remember that problem solving is a strategy that will work when you want to tackle practical problems or obstacles, which before might have seemed insurmountable. If you are finding it hard to problem solve around a particularly challenging issue, you may also find it helpful to consult a health care professional for advice or see a Clinical Psychologist or Psychotherapist for more in-depth therapy or counselling. Sometimes, when you feel overwhelmed by emotions, you may not be able to use the problem solving strategies explored in this chapter and during those times support that helps you address and acknowledge your emotions, may be more helpful to you.

# 12

## Visualising the Future

# INTRODUCTION

Your prognosis or chances for living well with HIV infection are better than they have ever been. However, the quality of your life on a daily basis is just as important as the number of years you will live. The more you are going to give your life meaning, the more you can hold a positive and enjoyable outlook and the greater your psychological well-being will be and your ability to withstand what life brings you.

We know that living with a chronic illness, such as HIV, can present challenges to building up a satisfying life. For example, drug treatments for HIV can make people, who are otherwise well, feel physically ill, because of their side effects. This may be a person's first experience of feeling unwell and not make sense to them, as they expected that drugs that are helpful to their health "should" not make them feel unwell. People who were diagnosed with HIV well before the advent of HAART have faced specific challenges in adapting to an increased life expectancy. A participant in a research study on the impact of "revival", or the experience of regaining health after ill health following the advent of the combination therapies, described his experiences, as follows:

> The weirdest thing for me now is that I am experiencing stress, because it now looks like I'm going to be living for a long time. You know, I'd said good-bye and I felt free from all these responsibilities that had to do with my career and so on… So, with me its almost as though the stress had really ended when I got really sick, because I had reached this kind of coming to terms. But now it has started up again, when I've gotten healthier. And that's the most perverse thing in the world…

It can be difficult to gain a sense of how to move forward in your life with HIV. In this chapter we offer some suggestions on how to build a life worth living with HIV by exploring with you how to take stock and visualize a fulfilling future.

### SELF-MONITORING: A CHANCE TO CHECK-IN WITH YOURSELF ● *the law of attraction* ( 1 ) *Have you ever heard of 'The Law of Attraction'? Although it is not a scientifically proven concept, it can be traced back in time. Basically it means that by knowing what you want or need, visualising it clearly and focusing your energy on it, you can be more receptive to creating and manifesting it in your life. (2) Try it out! Be mindful of your wishes. Develop a strong enthusiasm for that which you want in your life; know definitely what it is that you want and can achieve; ask for it in simple concise language; believe in the possibility of accomplishment; think about it and see yourself in the finished picture; feel gratitude for it; and lastly, feel expectancy for it and train yourself to live in a happy state of expectancy! At the very least it is a positive way of thinking! It could be very helpful to write your wishes down in your diary, notebook or on a sheet of paper, so that you can check in with them regularly and strengthen your desire for them.*

PART
A

PART
B

PART
C

# THE PAST AND THE PRESENT

Before you start any planning, it is important to reflect upon where you have got to now in your life. Did you put your life on hold, since your HIV diagnosis? What changes happened in your life when you learned of your diagnosis? Now is the time to evaluate the changes, think about the positive steps you would like to make and set up a plan of action. Some of these questions about your past might help you understand what has changed about your life since the diagnosis and what you might like to be different:

- Has my life changed much since being diagnosed HIV positive?
- What did my ambitions used to be and can I still achieve them?
- Have I changed my future plans, since being diagnosed with HIV?
- If so, does this make sense?
- Do I feel that the consequences of being HIV positive have stopped some of my plans from occurring? In what way?
- Has HIV made me want to gain more out of my life and make some positive changes?

Then you might like to think about now, the present, and ask yourself these questions:

- What am I doing with my life now that I am living with HIV?
- What ambitions do I now have?
- What ambitions would I like to cultivate?
- Where would I like to see myself in the future?
- What would I like to be doing five or ten years from now?

PART
A

PART
B

PART
C

# IDENTIFYING VALUES:
# WHAT I WANT MY LIFE TO STAND FOR?

What we "value" or regard as important to us, can enable us to make satisfying choices about how we want to live our lives. We all have values, but it is sometimes a matter of asking ourselves what they are as we may have lost sight of them.

Values are different from goals in a number of ways. They are deeply held and operate over very long time frames. They are not dependent on things being present in your life. For example, the value of being a caring partner is not dependent on having a partner. Sometimes people fall into the trap of saying: "if only I had a partner, then I would be happy", or: "if only I didn't suffer from anxiety, then I would be happy". If you believe that attaining goals is the key to life satisfaction this can lead to frustration and unhappiness by constantly reminding you of what you are missing in your life? Like a mirage, goals can seem elusive and when you think one is reached, a new one usually pops up quite quickly to keep you yearning. Values by contrast represent what is important to you. They are about something that you hold deeply inside yourself and they are unique to you as an individual and can keep you going in times of difficulty. Goals can be useful though, if they lead to action based on your values. To illustrate this, please read the following example.

PART A
PART B
PART C

*Paul* moved to the UK four years ago from abroad and was dissatisfied with his life mainly because of the absence of a satisfying job. He had been doing the same job for four years. A job he didn't like and which bored him, but he was earning enough to live off comfortably. Recently he was diagnosed HIV positive and began asking himself what he was doing with his life. He felt that it was important for his employment situation to change, but before this he thought about what he wanted his life to stand for in relation to his work. This included the type of work and his attraction to it, as well as, the values he would like to bring to it (e.g. in terms of his consciousness, feeling some social connection and that the work *provided something of worth to society). He then set goals in relation to his values, such as, visiting career advisers, obtaining information about course funding etc. He was soon doing something he liked, but more importantly also something he valued and that seemed to make a worthwhile contribution to society.*

Another way to identify values is to think about how you would like to be remembered 100 years from now. Pretend that a biographer is writing an epitaph about you. What would you like it to say? How would you like to be remembered?

Paul's epitaph, before he was diagnosed might have read something like: "spent his life wondering whether he could make something of it and died without an answer", whereas following his diagnosis it could read: "made a real difference in his job, did something he felt was worthwhile and was well-liked amongst his colleagues".

In Figure (32) a range of life areas are specified. You could begin asking yourself what you would like your life to stand for in relation to them. What values do you hold in relation to your health, relationships, friendships and work?

SELF-MONITORING: A CHANCE TO CHECK-IN WITH YOURSELF * *visualisation ( 1 ) Figure (32), opposite, shows a chart upon which you can attempt to map out your future. Use the chart to write and consider your future possibilities. Make sure your responses to these questions include your career or vocation, health, family and friends, travel and so on. (2) It may seem hard to think about the future, especially ten years from now. But what is the harm in attempting to focus on where you want your life to go? We would like to encourage you to try and see your future life as*

## MY FUTURE

|  | 1 YEAR | 5 YEARS | 10 YEARS |
|---|---|---|---|
| Health and well being |  |  |  |
| Home |  |  |  |
| Friends |  |  |  |
| Family |  |  |  |
| Leisure |  |  |  |
| Career / vocation |  |  |  |
| Other |  |  |  |

**Fig. 32** My future

clearly as possible. When you have developed a clear vision of your
future, try and hold onto this image. Get an internally felt sense of:
How you will be feeling, who will be around, what you will be doing
and how healthy you will be. Once you have really a sense of this try
to anchor or hold onto these feelings by recalling the feelings of well
being associated with them, or an image they create in your mind. It
could be very helpful to write your visualized feelings down in your

*diary, notebook or on a sheet of paper, so that you can return to these frequently and strengthen or expand on them.*

While attempting to think about Figure (32), you may come across some problems in doing so, particularly if you are depressed or anxious. Below are some common traps people may fall into that prevents them from truly going with what they value:

OWNERSHIP OF VALUES. Doing things that are more about others than yourself is unlikely to sustain you. You can ask yourself the question: "imagine if X (parent, partner, friend, therapist etc) never found out about Y (course, job, volunteering, holiday, etc) would I still be doing it? Do things for yourself, even if someone else may not value it.

BETTER THE DEVIL YOU KNOW. If things haven't worked out in the past, people are often afraid to try again as it seems too risky. If this is the case, you might say: "things are not good now, but if I try I could be even worse off". What value does this position reflect? Maybe "Spent his life being too afraid to try." Do attempt things that may not have worked for you before because at a different time and under different circumstances they might work better, especially if you do them out of a position that truly reflects your own values and not the values of others. For example, if you really wanted a particular job and did not get it in the past, this does not mean that you should not apply for another, interesting job again. Don't give up on trying new things, which might be rewarding for you, because you are frightened of making mistakes.

WHAT OTHER PEOPLE SAY WILL INFLUENCE YOUR CONFIDENCE AND MOTIVATION. Listen to advice, but remember that some people

PART
A

PART
B

PART
C

may have vested interests in you not changing or may not appreciate what your values are. Do things because they are right for you. This is your life and only you can know what feels right and true to you. You are the one, like any one of us, who has to ultimately live his or her life and is accountable and responsible for the decisions you make. Therefore, it is important that you make your decisions, according to your own highest values. You can never feel truly confident and motivated if the things you do don't reflect your own values, but the values of others. It is therefore important for you to follow whatever reflects the values of your own sense of Self.

If you see life like getting to the top of a mountain, it will be easier to climb if you do not struggle against it and accept it, with its ups and downs and ravines, just like climbing a real mountain. Life will often bring challenges, which you may not have anticipated and didn't expect in that way. If you can shift your position from: "If only I wasn't anxious, or HIV positive I would be happy!" to "I am happy and HIV positive and anxious. I accept it all – but will build on it and live my life as positively as I can!".

PART
A

PART
B

PART
C

## SO HOW CAN I MAKE MY FUTURE HAPPEN?

Addressing many of the issues covered in this book will help you lay good foundations for living a positive life with HIV. We have offered you techniques and strategies that can work for you – your task will be to find and try out those, which suit you best at any given point in time. The following tips relate to the psychological, problem-solving, support seeking and acceptance methods advocated in this book and will help achieve the realities of a future you may want.

# SOME FINAL KEY TIPS
# TO LIVING CONFIDENTLY WITH HIV

1 *Understand the effects of HIV and how to live with it. Do accept that your life is different since your HIV diagnosis, but the extent to how different it can be, depends on how you deal with it. Allow yourself to see this as an opportunity to live your life as fully as you can, according to your own highest values. You may find, if you do this, that you feel more fulfilled, happy and true to yourself than you have ever felt before your HIV diagnosis.*

2 *Engage in a healthy lifestyle and negotiate your needs with your health care system.*

3 *Seek social support where necessary – why do some things on your own when there are many good people, agencies and services eager to assist? Be clear and honest with the people potentially assisting you, about what you really need, rather than assuming that they will know.*

4 *Disclose HIV where appropriate and with confidence and communicate your HIV status, where and when appropriate so that you can receive the right support from the right people.*

5 *Choose to have safer sexual relationships, but remember to disclose your HIV status to important partners and use safer sex.*

6 *Recognize, accept and manage your emotions in relation to the HIV. Allow yourself to try some of the methods introduced in this*

book, but seek extra professional help from an appropriately trained Psychotherapist or a Clinical Psychologist, should you feel that you need more in-depth, individually tailored support. Don't hold back on additional psychological help, should you feel you need it.

7 Problem solve dilemmas and think of small steps that you can take to achieve your valued goals. Be patient and kind to yourself and recognize that each step, however small it may seem, is movement toward a possible solution. Recognize your ability to positively bring change into your life.

8 Keep making future plans as your life need not be unsatisfying when living with HIV. Only you can create a valued future within your own life – allow yourself the possibility of working toward this.

PART A

PART B

PART C

# CONCLUSION – THE FUTURE!

The aim of this self-help book is to help you to make your future worthwhile while living with HIV. We are fortunate, following the advent of combination therapies that those living with HIV can now focus on living as well as they can, because having a chronic condition means you do have a future. When and where available, HAART treatments improve and sustain life, even if there is still no cure for now. Any uncertainty this may cause can be accepted if you are living a life you still value. Having plans for the long term is now very possible. Not only may such plans improve your general health, but also it makes plain good sense to be proactive in your life and take part in creating your future.

The more you can visualise a valued future and the clearer and detailed the vision, and the more energy you put into it, the more likely you'll be able to achieve it. This is really important, because the stronger you are able to imagine your future, literally developing a felt sense of it, the more likely you will bring it into reality. A word of caution though: remember, everyone has a future, but no one knows quite what it will be like. It has been found that visualization is a very powerful tool, but be mindful that just as much as positive visualization of your future may attract positive experiences, so might negative visualization bring about negative experiences. As an old saying goes: "be careful of what you wish for, as it may actually happen!". Therefore become aware of the quality of your thoughts and feelings and work toward a positive future, which is in line with your own value system.

This book contains many practical tips and techniques to enable you to plan positively for the future. Remember, you are in a position to influence what happens tomorrow and in ten years from now.

We hope that this book has provided you with new insights into your life and some ways forward. There are many things you can do, people and supports you can seek out, and possible changes you can make, which can all lead to a rewarding future. This book has attempted to put across ways of living confidently with HIV and to help you build a life worth living. The key character in all of this is you. We wish you well in your journey.

# Appendix
# & Resources,
# Glossary,
# Index

## ALCOHOLICS ANONYMOUS

UK National Helpline 0845 769 7555
The General Service Board of Alcoholics
Anonymous (Great Britain) Ltd.
Registered Office: PO Box 1,
10 Toft Green, York, YO1 7NJ
www. alcoholics-anonymour.org.uk

## BLUE STALLION PUBLICATIONS

Specialist publisher for psychological
self-help material. Books can be ordered
through: www.oxdev.co.uk and www.
mybookstation.co.uk  Tel: 01452 302 670

## HIV i-Base

Produces publications and information for
people with HIV
3rd Floor East, Thrale House, 44-46
Southwark St, London SE1 1UN
HIV Treatment information for healthcare
professionals and HIV+ people. Avoiding and
managing side effects. (May 2008)
info@i-base.org.uk
www.i-base.info
General enquiries: admin@i-base.org.uk
Tel: 0207 407 8488
Treatment information phone line: mon-wed
12-4 pm Tel: 0808 8006013

## NARCOTICS ANONYMOUS

Websites: www.ukna.org
NAHelpline@ukna.org
UK National Helpline: 0845 373 3366 or
0208 77300009

## Body and Soul HIV/AIDS Charity London UK

Supporting children, teenagers, women and
heterosexual men with HIV/AIDS
Tel: 0207 3837678
Website: www.bodyandsoulcharity.org

## BRITISH ASSOCIATION OF BEHAVIOURAL AND COGNITIVE PSYCHOTHERAPY (BABCP)

British Association for Behavioural and
Cognitive Psychotherapy
Victoria Buildings, 9-13 Silver Street, Bury
BL9 0EU
Tel: 0161 797 4484
Fax: 0161 797 2670
Email: babcp@babcp.com
Website: www.babcp.com

## BRITISH ASSOCIATION OF PSYCHOTHERAPISTS (BAP)

British Association of Psychotherapists
37 Mapesbury Rd, London NW2 4 HJ
Tel: 0208 452 9823
Email: mail@bap-psychotherapy.org
Website: www.bap-psychotherapy.org

## BRITISH ASSOCIATION FOR SEXUAL AND RELATIONSHIP THERAPY (BASRT)

Tel: 020 8543 2707
Email: info@basrt.org.uk
Website: www.basrt.org.uk

## BRITISH HIV ASSOCIATION

British (BHIVA) pregnancy and treatment
guidelines
Website: www.bhiva.org
BHIVA Secretariat, Mediscript Ltd,
1 Mountview Court, 310 Friern Barnet Lane
London. N20 0LD United Kingdom
Tel: +44 (0)20 8369 5380

**BRITISH PSYCHOLOGICAL SOCIETY**
(BPS) British Psychological Society
St. Andrew's House, 48 Princess Road East,
Leicester LE1 7DR
Tel: 0116 254 9568
Website: www.bps.org.uk

**CHILDREN'S HIV ASSOCIATION (CHIVA)**
CHIVA Secretariat, Mediscript Ltd
1 Mountview Court, 310 Friern Barnet Lane
London N20 0LD
Tel: +44 (0)20 8446 8898
Fax: +44 (0)20 8446 9194
Email: chiva@chiva.org.uk

**CHILDREN and YOUNG PEOPLE
with HIV**

Lwin, R., Duggan, C. & Gibb, D.M. (1994).
*HIV and AIDS in Children. A Guide for
The Family.* Great Ormond Street Hospital.
John Brown Ltd: Great Britain.

Elizabeth Lewis (2001). *Afraid to Say:
The needs and views of young people
living with HIV/AIDS.* National Children's
Bureau. Impress Print: Corby.

**CITIZENS ADVICE BUREAU (CAB)**
Registered office: Myddelton House, 115-123
Pentonville Road, London, N1 9LZ.
Website: www.citizenadvice.org.uk

**ELTON JOHN AIDS FOUNDATION**
A charity that supports people with HIV/AIDS
worldwide through prevention, grants and
projects to reduce stigma and discrimination.
P.O. Box 17139, Beverly Hills,
CA 90209-3139
Elton John AIDS Foundation, 584 Broadway,
Suite 907, New York. NY 10012
www.ejaf.org

**Embrace Community Support Centre**
Community Support Centre, a registered
charity, aims to relieve poverty among
disadvantaged groups, including refugees,
asylum seekers and migrants through the
provision of information, advice and guidance
on welfare benefits, housing, immigration,
education and training, health-related issues
and conducts research as necessary.
Selby Centre, Selby Road, London N17 8JL
Tel: 0208 801 92224
Website: www.embraceuk.org

**Family PLANNING ASSOCIATION**
UK office, 50 Featherstone Street
London EC1Y 8QU
Tel: 020 7608 5240
Fax: 0845 123 2349
National Helpline 0845 122 8600 (Open
Monday to Friday, 9am to 6pm).
Website: www.fpa.org.uk

**HEALTH FOR ASYLUM SEEKERS &
REFUGEES PORTAL (HARP)**
A web site focussing on mental health and
well-being issues as they affect asylum
seekers and refugees.
Website: http://mentalhealth.harpweb.org.uk

**HEALTH PROFESSIONS COUNCIL**
(HPC) UK-wide regulator for Practitioner
Psychologists, such as Clinical or Counselling
Psychologists, and other Healthcare

Professionals, which was created with a special remit to protect the public. The HPC keeps on online register of all healthcare professionals regulated through them.
Park House, 184 Kennington Park Road
London SE11 4BU
Tel: 0207 840 9802
Website: www.hpc-uk.org

## LONDON LESBIAN AND GAY SWITCHBOARD

A 24-hour, seven-days-a-week helpline that offers you a range of services, including advice about your sexual health.
London Lesbian & Gay Switchboard
PO Box 7324, London N1 9QS
Helpline: 020 7837 7324
Office: 020 7837 6768
Fax: 020 7837 7300
Email: admin@llgs.org.uk

## MINDFULNESS RESOURCES

Kabat-Zinn, J. (1994). *Wherever you go, there you are: Mindfulness meditation in everyday life*. New York: Hyperion.

Kabat-Zinn, J. (1990). *Full Catastrophe Living: Using the wisdom of your body and mind to face stress, pain, and illness*. New York: Dell Publishing.

Segal, Z.V., Williams, J.M. & Teasdale, J.D. (2002) *Mindfulness based cognitive therapy for depression*. New York: Guildford Press.

Guided body scan and other guided

meditation tapes can be purchased from The Oxford Stress and Trauma Centre on: www.oxdev.co.uk or www.mybookstation.co.uk

## NATIONAL ASSOCIATION FOR MENTAL HEALTH (MIND)

Information Line 0845 766 0163
Website: www.mind.org.uk

## NATIONAL AIDS HELPLINE (NAH)

A 24-hour, seven-days-a-week, free and confidential telephone service with advice about HIV, AIDS sexual health, local services, clinics and support services.
Tel: 0800 567 123 & 0800 555 777

## NAM and AIDSMAP

Provides information on HI/AIDS
Lincoln House, 1 Brixton Road
London SW9 6DE
Tel: 020 7840 0050
Email: info@nam.org.uk
Website: www.aidsmap.com

## NATIONAL AIDS TRUST (NAT)

A charity dedicated to transforming societies response to HIV, providing advice, practical resources and campaigning for change.
London EC1V 9FR
Tel: 0207 814 6767
Email: info@nat.org.uk

## NATIONAL SEXUAL HEALTH HELPLINE

Tel: 0800 567 123

## THE OXFORD DEVELOPMENT CENTRE

Independent psychological therapy centre,

offering several different services, aimed at helping clients with a large variety of problems. This includes HIV+ and other chronic illness related difficulties and issues; specialist interventions for overcoming trauma; partner and couple's work; depression; addictions and most other psychological difficulties. Entirely private, confidential, non-NHS based service. Specialising in a holistic Positive Psychology approach, including Positive Growth Therapy (PGT), which seeks to promote each person's individual well-being, inner strength and growth and values each person as a unique human being. Appointments can be made directly with the service. Recognized by most major health insurance companies.

The Oxford Development Centre, includes: The Oxford Stress and Trauma Centre and Oxfordshire's Independent Psychology Service
47 High Street, Witney
Oxfordshire OX28 6JA
Tel. 01993 77 99 94 or 01993 77 90 77
Fax: 01993 77 94 99
Website: www.oxdev.co.uk

### POSITIVELY WOMEN
Provides support for women living with HIV by women living with HIV.
347-349 City Rd, London EC1V 1LR
Tel: 0207 713 0444
Website: www.positively. women.org.uk

### PROJECT FOR ADVICE, COUNSELLING AND EDUCATION (PACE)
Provides counselling, advocacy, groups, workshops, HIV prevention, employment advice, youthwork, and training. All staff and volunteers at PACE identify as gay or lesbian.
34 Hartham Rd, London N7 9JL
Tel: 020 7700 1323
Email: pace@dircon.co.uk
Website: www.pacehealth.org.uk

### RELATE
A national counselling organisation. It can put you in touch with their local branches. Relate offers confidential counselling to individuals and couples on relationship and sexual difficulties.
Tel: 01788 573 241
Website: www.relate.org.uk

### SEXUAL FUNCTIONING

📖 Zilbergeld, B. (1980). *Men and Sex.* London: Fontana.

📖 Milsten, R. & Slowinski, J. (1999). *The Sexual Male – Problems and Solutions. A Complete Medical and Psychological Guide to Lifelong Potency*

📖 Steward, E. & Spencer, P. (2002). *The V Book: A Doctor's Guide to Complete Vulvovaginal Health.* New York: Bantam

### THE SEXUAL DYSFUNCTION ASSOCIATION
Suite 301. Emblem House
London Bridge Hospital
27 Tooley Street, London SE1 2PR
Helpline 0870 774 3571

Email: info@sda.uk.net

Website: www.sda.uk.net

**STONEWALL**

Equality and Justice for Lesbians, Gay Men and Bisexuals

Tower Building, York Road

London SE1 7NX

Telephone: 020 7593 1850

Info Line: 08000 50 20 20

Fax: 020 7593 1877

Minicom: 020 7633 0759

Email: info@stonewall.org.uk

**TERRENCE HIGGINS TRUST**

52-54 Grays Inn Road

London WC1X 8JU

Tel: 020 7831 0330

THT Direct Helpline: 0845 12 21 200

(Monday-Friday 10am-10pm, and Saturday & Sunday 12pm – 6pm)

Email: info@tht.org.uk

Website: www.tht.org.uk

**UNITED KINGDOM COUNCIL FOR PSYCHOTHERAPY (UKCP)**

UK Council for Psychotherapy

2nd Floor Edward House

2 Wakley Street, London EC1V 7LT

Tel: 020 7014 9955

Fax: 020 7014 9977

E-mail: info@psychotherapy.org.uk

Website: www.ukcp.org.uk

These books can be purchased from www.mybookstation.co.uk

# GLOSSARY

**ASYMPTOMATIC** When a person who is HIV positive has no HIV related symptoms and is feeling generally well.

$CD_4$ A key cell which co-ordinates the body's fight against infection.

**COMBINATION THERAPY** Taking more than one anti-HIV drug at a time to attack HIV.

**COMPLIANCE** Someone's ability to take the drugs they have been given exactly as instructed.

**DISEASE PROGRESSION** The worsening of disease.

**DRUG REGIME** How a drug needs to be taken e.g. three times a day with food.

**IMMUNE SYSTEM** The body's system for fighting infection.

**PERIPHERAL NEUROPATHY** Painful tingling of feet, and sometimes in hands.

**RELAPSE** To become ill again after recovering from being unwell.

**RESISTANCE** When the drugs used to attack HIV don't have an effect anymore because the virus has changed its structure.

**SIDE EFFECTS** Unwanted symptoms caused by a particular medicine rather than a disease.

**SYMPTOMS** A sensation or change in the body's normal functions which is usually linked to a particular disease.

**UNDETECTABLE VIRAL LOAD** Where there are not enough HIV particles in a blood sample for the viral load test to count. It does not mean that you do not have any HIV in your blood.

**WHITE BLOOD CELLS** The cells that make up the immune system.

# INDEX

# DONATION FORM

Included in the purchase price of this book is a donation of £1.50, which Blue Stallion Publications will automatically forward to The Elton John AIDS Foundation.

## Gift Aid

If you are a UK taxpayer, you can increase this donation, at no extra cost to yourself, by 25%, simply by providing your address details, including postcode, as proof of your UK residence. Blue Stallion Publications will then apply for Gift Aid on your behalf.

First name:

Second name:

Address:

Postcode

## Further Donation

If you would like to make a further donation, please complete the back of this form on the next page.

>

# DONATION FORM cont.

I would like to donate to...                                    £

## Elton John AIDS Foundation

## Terrence Higgings Trust

**A charity of your choice:**
name:
address:

Total [                ]

All donations will be forwarded quarterly to the charities.

## Payment method

Credit card/Switch                              Cheque

Card number:
Expiry date:
Issue Number (Switch)
Security Number:

## Please send your completed form to:

Blue Stallion Publications, Unit 5, Shepherd Road
Industrial Estate, Cole Avenue, Gloucester, GL2 5HL